BRAIN BASICS®: SLEEP
A GUIDE TO UNDERSTANDING SLEEP

PART OF THE BRAIN BASICS® SERIES

by
Robert A. Williams, M.D.

Brain Basics®: Sleep is a book to enhance the basic understanding of sleep. *Brain Basics®: Sleep* is not meant to be a comprehensive academic textbook. To simplify and to amplify understanding, models and metaphors are used. Repetition of concepts are used to enhance understanding.

It is not the purpose of *Brain Basics®: Sleep* to provide an in-depth examination of any of the sleep disorders described, but to provide a basic framework of understanding.

Published by:
Biological Psychiatry Institute, Ltd.
5133 North Central Avenue, Suite 107
Phoenix, Arizona 85012

ISBN: 978-9754599-1-1

Printed in the United States of America

"The beginning of health is sleep."

It is obvious from the over-the-counter sales of sleep medicines that insomnia is a common problem. One might ask, "What is the problem?" The insomniac states, "I can't sleep!" The answer commonly is taking a pill for insomnia and you'll feel better. One might also ask the question, "What should I do for a fever?" The inappropriate answer might be to take an antibiotic without knowing what is causing the fever. The correct question is where is the infection or is there an infection at all? Likewise, insomnia is a symptom. And, the appropriate question is what is causing the insomnia?

After reading **Brain Basics®: Sleep,** you will better understand the mechanisms of sleep and the causes of insomnia. And, hopefully, the information in **Brain Basics®: Sleep** will help you understand any sleep problem.

Some of the questions answered in **Brain Basics®: Sleep** are as follows:

1. What is sleep?
2. What are the fundamentals of sleep?
3. What are the mechanisms of sleep disorders?
4. How do sleep disorder mechanisms relate to the five definitions of sleep disorders as described in the Diagnostic Statistical Manual IV-R?
5. How do sleep disorders relate to other medical disorders?

Williams Brain Model

Three Steps To Get To Sleep

Sleep is a process that creates neurotransmitter gas and energy that runs the brain engine the next day.

There are three steps needed to get to sleep.

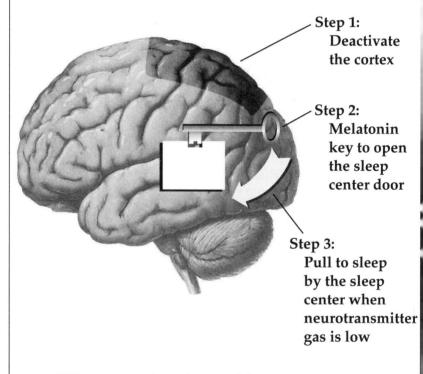

Step 1:
Deactivate the cortex

Step 2:
Melatonin key to open the sleep center door

Step 3:
Pull to sleep by the sleep center when neurotransmitter gas is low

When a patient is unable to get to sleep he will complain of "insomnia."

Williams Brain Model
Three Steps To Get Restorative Sleep

Sleep is the process that creates neurotransmitter gas and energy that runs the brain engine the next day. Restorative sleep occurs when a person awakes feeling rested and feeling well and has a sense of well-being.

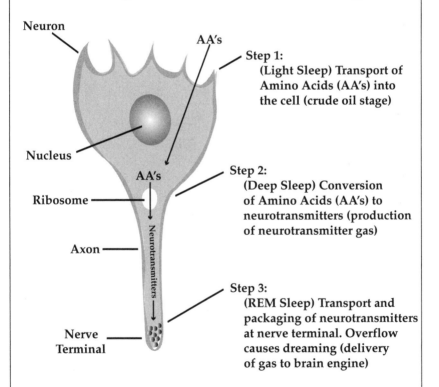

Neuron

AA's

Nucleus

AA's

Ribosome

Axon

Neurotransmitters

Nerve Terminal

Step 1:
(Light Sleep) Transport of Amino Acids (AA's) into the cell (crude oil stage)

Step 2:
(Deep Sleep) Conversion of Amino Acids (AA's) to neurotransmitters (production of neurotransmitter gas)

Step 3:
(REM Sleep) Transport and packaging of neurotransmitters at nerve terminal. Overflow causes dreaming (delivery of gas to brain engine)

When a person does not get Restorative Sleep, they complain of daytime "tiredness" and have propensity to fall asleep (daytime hypersomnolance).

Brain Basics®: Sleep is divided into four sections.

The first section is the Introduction and the last section is the Summary.

The second section is What is Needed to Get to Sleep? There are three steps needed to get to sleep. There are three chapters in Section 2 corresponding to the three steps to get to sleep.

The third section is What is Needed to Get Restorative Sleep? There are three steps that are needed to get restorative sleep. There are three chapters in Section 3 corresponding to the three steps needed to get restorative sleep.

Normal sleep is based on getting to sleep, staying asleep and getting restorative sleep. Therefore, it is proposed that if a person understands the three steps needed to get to sleep and the three steps needed to get restorative sleep, that any sleep problem can be understood.

TABLE OF CONTENTS

PREFACE

The purpose of *Brain Basics®: Sleep* is to enhance any interested party's knowledge and understanding of sleep. Metaphors and concepts are provided for heuristic purposes (to enhance understanding). There are terms used in a conceptual sense, not to be confused with the literal sense. For instance, "tank" is used as one would think of a gas tank. There are no "tanks" in the brain, but "tank" is used to mean a potential physical reserve of a substance such as a neurotransmitter "tank" or a melatonin "tank." Another example of a metaphor is melatonin "key." There is no literal lock and key in the brain. I have found the use of metaphors to greatly help patients understand brain processes including sleep. Poetic license is frequently used in *Brain Basics®: Sleep* as well as oversimplification for heuristic purposes.

Sleep is not only necessary for normal brain function, sleep is necessary for life. Severe sleep deprivation will result in death. Mild sleep deprivation results in tiredness, irritability and attention deficits. Moderate sleep deprivation results in all the symptoms of mild sleep deprivation plus dysfunction of generators of behavior that a person is vulnerable to; such as depression, anger or rage, obsessiveness or anxiety. Severe sleep deprivation results in all those symptoms in moderate sleep deprivation plus psychosis, frontal lobe syndrome (confusion, impulsivity, poor judgment and signs of catatonia) or "brain fog," inability to perform tasks and brain stem instability that can result in death. All levels of sleep deprivation affect the immune system adversely.

Why is it desirable to go to sleep on time or at a desired clock time? The main reason is the world works during the day and sleeps at night. Therefore, if a person cannot sleep at night and forces himself to get up in the morning, he will be sleep deprived.

SECTION 1

INTRODUCTION TO SLEEP

Chapter 1

Introduction

*"Care keeps his watch in every old man's eye,
and where care lodges, sleep will never lie."*

ROMEO & JULIET
ACT II, SC. 3

"Anxiety can disrupt sleep."

ROBERT A. WILLIAMS, M.D.

The brain has two main states: awake and asleep. Awake states are for the purpose of creating human behavior under the control of the frontal lobes. Sleep states are for the purpose of restoring the brain under control of the sleep center. Sleep restores neurotransmitter and energy reserves so the brain can function during the awake state.

Outwardly a person may appear as if he/she is unconscious or sleeping, but the person sleeping is far from unconscious. For instance, a person sleeping has the capacity to experience pain as compared to a person under anesthesia who cannot. Or, a person sleeping can easily be aroused while a person in a coma cannot. Or, a person can act as if asleep while fully awake. Sleep is a unique internal state for the purpose of restoring brain reserves.

The state of being asleep is measured by polysomnography. Adequacy of sleep is measured subjectively by the individual. The basic question in terms of adequacy of sleep is "Does the individual feel restored (refreshed), feel well and function well after a night's sleep?"

The brain is a behavioral engine that runs on neurotransmitter gas. During restorative sleep, the neurotransmitter gas tank is filled up. Sleep disorders occur when the brain runs out of gas and the brain fails in its usual awake capacities.

The region of the brain most sensitive to the lack of gas is our executive function in the frontal lobes. Executive function is a gas-guzzling part of the brain. Executive function is the driver of the brain engine. When persons are sleep deprived, they tend to have executive function failure including decreased capacity to modulate behavior (i.e., irritability), decreased capacity to concentrate and perform tasks, impulsivity and poor judgment. Accidents may be the result of sleep deprivation. Sleep deprivation contributes to road rage (i.e., frontal lobe incapacity to modulate anger).

There are three objectives in the treatment of psychiatric disorders. These are **The Williams' Three Wells,** which define biological *stability* in the brain.

1. *Sleep Well.* A patient needs gas (i.e., neurotransmitters) for the brain machine (personality) to run during the awake state (i.e., gas is delivered to the engine).
2. *Feel Well.* Personality is the overlapping matrix of all the generators of behavior in the brain. Feeling well means there is no generator of behavior interfering with personality behavior such as depression and/or anxiety. Personality is the brain machine.
3. *Function Well.* Executive function involves modulation of generators of behavior, coping, interpersonal communication, planning and execution of tasks and decision making.[1] Executive function is the driver of the brain engine to reach goals.

The importance of sleep in a psychiatric practice cannot be overemphasized. The need to sleep well is a basic need for normal brain function. The first step in evaluating biological stability is the evaluation of sleep. Without the neurotransmitter gas to run the brain engine, the brain engine will sputter.

There is evidence that supports a common pathophysiologic pathway between sleep disorders and psychiatric disorders. It is thought that low neurotransmitter levels in the synaptic cleft (space between two brain cells where neurotransmitters cross to communicate) relate to depression. A 42-month study of patients with insomnia[2] showed a twelve-fold increase of depression compared to a controlled population (Figure 1-1). I propose that the main function of sleep is to fill up the neurotransmitter gas tank to run the brain engine. If patients have non-restorative sleep, the availability of neurotransmitters is low. Low neurotransmitters mimic what we see with primary depressions. The actions of most antidepressants is to block the re-uptake of neurotransmitters and thereby increase the availability of neurotransmitters in the synaptic cleft. Thirty to 40 percent of patients with treatment-resistant depression have sleep disorders. When the sleep disorder is corrected, the patient becomes more treatment responsive. Antidepressants work better when the neurotransmitter loads are more available to block the re-uptake thereof.

Figure 1-1: Brain Cell Mechanisms in Disease

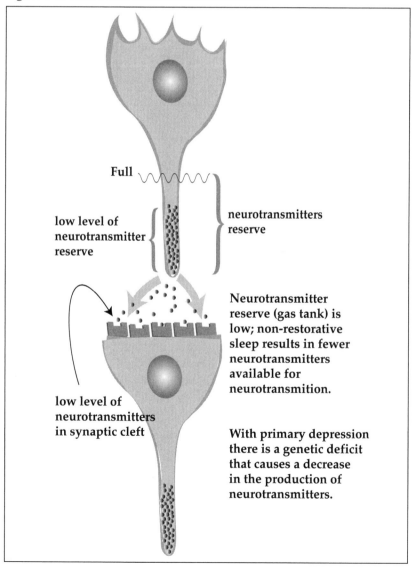

Full

low level of neurotransmitter reserve

neurotransmitters reserve

Neurotransmitter reserve (gas tank) is low; non-restorative sleep results in fewer neurotransmitters available for neurotransmition.

low level of neurotransmitters in synaptic cleft

With primary depression there is a genetic deficit that causes a decrease in the production of neurotransmitters.

Figure 1-2: Consequences of Insomnia: Risk of Psychiatric Disorders[3]

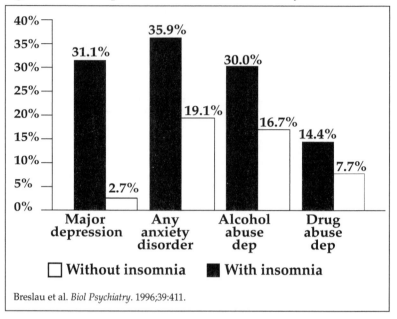

Breslau et al. *Biol Psychiatry*. 1996;39:411.

In the evaluation of a psychiatric patient, it is sometimes hard to sort out what causes a sleep problem, because psychiatric disorders in themselves cause sleep problems. In other words, there are times when it is hard to know cause and effect. For example, patients commonly have both depression and insomnia. The fundamental problem is did the depression cause insomnia or did the insomnia cause depression? Or, the depression and insomnia may occur independent of each other, but worsen the symptoms of each.

The main source of data in sorting out cause and effect is the patient's past history. For example, if a depressed patient has a normal history of sleep before getting depressed, and insomnia after getting depressed, it is reasonable to assume the sleep disorder is secondary to depression. Even though a sleep disorder is secondary to depression, the sleep disorder must be treated as a separate issue because insomnia worsens depression. When the depression resolves, the sleep disorder secondary to the depression resolves. If per chance, insomnia persists beyond the resolution of depression, the insomnia should be considered a separate problem.

Discongruity between symptoms of illness is sometimes seen. One form of brain failure is defined as a behavior cluster. The DSM IV* provides a behavioral cluster as seen in the major depression cluster. Note the fourth criteria for major depression is insomnia or hypersomnia nearly

*Diagnostic Statistical Manual IV-TR

every day. When a sleep problem is caused by depression it resolves within the treatment of depression.

Figure 1-3: Diagnostic Statistic Manual of Mental Disorders IV

■ **Criteria for Major Depressive Episode**

A. Five (or more) of the following symptoms have been present during the same 2-week period and represent a change from previous functioning; at least one of the symptoms is either (1) depressed mood or (2) loss of interest or pleasure.
Note: Do not include symptoms that are clearly due to a general medical condition, or mood-incongruent delusions or hallucinations.

  (1) depressed mood most of the day, nearly every day, as indicated by either subjective report (e.g., feels sad or empty) or observation made by others (e.g., appears tearful). **Note:** In children and adolescents, can be irritable mood.

  (2) markedly diminished interest or pleasure in all, or almost all, activities most of the day, nearly every day (as indicated by either subjective account or observation made by others).

  (3) significant weight lost when not dieting or weight gain (e.g., a change of more than 5% of body weight in a month), or decrease or increase in appetite nearly every day. **Note:**In children, consider failure to make expected weight gains.

  (4) *insomnia or hypersomnia nearly every day (sleep problem is a symptom of depression).*

  (5) psychomotor agitation or retardation nearly every day (observable by others, not merely subjective feelings of restlessness or being slowed down).

  (6) fatigue or loss of energy nearly every day.

  (7) feelings of worthlessness or excessive or inappropriate guilt (which may be delusional) nearly every day (not merely self-reproach or guilt about being sick).

  (8) diminished ability to think or concentrate or indecisiveness, nearly every day (either by subjective account or as observed by others).

  (9) recurrent thoughts of death (not just fear of dying), recurrent suicidal ideation without a specific plan, or a suicide attempt or a specific plan for committing suicide.

B. The symptoms do not meet criteria for a Mixed Episode (see p. 335).

C. The symptoms cause clinically significant distress or impairment in social, occupational, or other important areas of functioning.

D. The symptoms are not due to the direct physiological effects of a substance (e.g., a drug of abuse, a medication) or a general medical condition (e.g., hypothyroidism).

E. The symptoms are not better accounted for by Bereavement, (i.e., after the loss of a loved one,) the symptoms persist for longer than 2 months or are characterized by marked functional impairment, morbid preoccupation with worthlessness, suicidal ideation, psychotic symptoms, or psychomotor retardation.

American Psychiatric Association: *Diagnostic and Statistical Manual of Mental Disorders,* Fourth Edition, Text Revision. Washington, DC, American Psychiatric Association, 2000, pg. 356.

Usually, the behavior cluster symptoms worsen as a group as the depressive illness worsens. In other words, mild illness produces mild depression and mild insomnia. Or, severe depression illness produces severe depression and severe insomnia. In the case where depression is mild and the sleep disorder is severe, one suspects from the incongruity, that the sleep disorder is separate from the depression.

The other case is where a patient has a long history (perhaps weeks or months) of insomnia and develops depression. The major focus is on the diagnosis and treatment of the sleep disorder. Of course, as a separate issue, the depression is treated. After the sleep disorder is treated, one would expect the depression to resolve without the use of antidepressants. If the depression persists beyond the time the sleep disorder is stable, then depression is considered as a separate problem.

We observe that biological depression can be the consequence of many medical conditions such as hypothyroidism, multiple sclerosis, strokes, sleep disorders, vitamin deficiency, lung disorders and a whole host of others. Once the abnormal neuro-mechanisms or pathways have been activated to produce biological depression, the brain is changed forever. It is called kindling. Kindling refers to the ever-increasing ease of activating abnormal neuro-mechanisms with each sequential psychiatric relapse. It is likened to the kindling in starting a fire. The more kindling you have, the easier it is to start a fire.

In the case of sleep disorders activating depression, the reversibility of the depression would be determined with time. After the maximum treatment of the sleep disorder, the antidepressants that were used to treat depression may be tapered over a one- or two-month period. One would observe for a depressive relapse and reutilize the antidepressants as needed.

Chronic sleep disorders cause structural changes in the brain. The chronic metabolic stress on the brain from a chronic sleep problem causes brain cells to shrink and shrivel. When a chronic sleep disorder is diagnosed and treated, the patient will not have 100 percent immediate improvement. The chronic effects of a sleep disorder after treatment will improve at a rate of 10 to 20 percent per month. Or, it can take nearly a year to reverse the effects of a chronic sleep disorder. I give words of encouragement to my patients, "A slow recovery does not mean you won't get a full recovery."

There are several principles of Biological Psychiatry present in *Brain Basics®: Sleep*. I will review some of the relevant biological principles.

1. Generators of behavior are systems of neurons (i.e., brain cells) that have a common function. Examples of generators of behavior are:
   • memory generator of behavior
   • mood generator of behavior
   • sleep generator of behavior
2. The overlapping matrix of all the generators of behavior create personality behavior. It is the vast array of association fibers that connects the various generators of behavior. The connections ultimately create the overlapping matrix of behavior.
3. When a generator of behavior fails, it produces a predictable behavior cluster.
4. The behavior cluster involves the failed generator of behavior itself and the effects on other generators of behavior.

If a patient has an inherent vulnerability for a sleep disorder, major depression may present with a dominant feature of a sleep disorder. 35 percent[4] of sleep disorder referrals are found to have a psychiatric cause such as major depression.

Figure 1-4: William Brain Model showing production of clinical syndrome

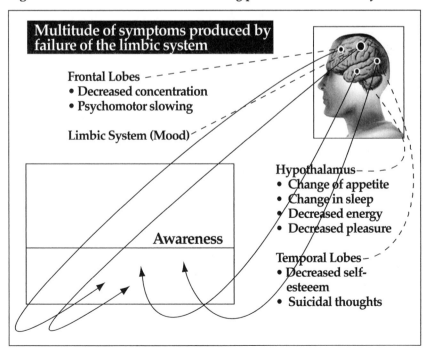

Illness is defined as an inherently vulnerable generator of behavior that has the capacity to produce behavior independent of normal personality behavior that interferes with normal functioning.

Sleep disorders produce obsessive thoughts about wanting to sleep and a profound sense of tiredness along with executive function dysfunction, depression, memory disturbances, anxiety and substance abuse that clearly interfere with how a person feels and functions. Therefore, sleep disorders are illnesses of the brain.

The subjective consequences of a sleep disturbance depend on the mechanism that is causing the sleep problem. For instance, if the problem involves getting and/or staying asleep, the patient complains of insomnia. The patient knows "if I could just get to sleep or stay asleep, then I would feel rested." The focus of treatment is on getting the patient asleep and keeping him asleep.

The following is an example of major depression caused by limbic system failure.

A 35-year-old married patient with one 10-year-old son starts to get progressive depression over a 2-month period. Her mother had depression at age 40. Her physical exam and laboratory values were normal. The patient satisfied the DSM IV criteria for depression, all nine out of nine criteria. The four treatment considerations are:
1. Survival—prevent suicide
2. Treat symptoms—treat insomnia as a separate issue
3. Treat underlying depression
4. Prevent relapse

Note: Sleep disturbance may be a symptom of depression or even the presenting complaint of major depression.

Note: It is not uncommon that a problem in one part of the brain affects other parts of the brain. Lack of sleep or sleep deprivation causes many brain problems as well as other physical problems.

Brain problems include:
1. Frontal lobe problems
   a. Reduced capacity to plan and execute tasks
   b. Reduced attention
   c. Increased impulsiveness
   d. Reduced capacity to modulate other generators of behavior (i.e., emotional over-reactivity)
   e. Reduced capacity to cope with stress
   f. Reduced capacity for judgement

2. Limbic problems include:
   a. Depression
   b. Reduced memory

3. Hypothalamic problems and anxiety include:
   a. Reduced energy and motivation
   b. Reduced sexual desire
   c. Increased appetite and weight (obesity)
   d. Decreased capacity for pleasure

4. Brain stem problems include:
   a. Anxiety
   b. Increased blood pressure and increased pulse
   c. Increased arrythmias
   d. Coronary vasospams
   e. Pulmonary hypertension

Profound consequences of insomnia affect executive function which cause grave deficiencies in the capacity to function. Executive function in the frontal lobes has many purposes. The following is a list of executive functions that are disrupted by insomnia:

1. Choose where one wants to focus on awareness.
2. Modulate specific generators of behavior. For example if you are nervous, calm down.
3. Use of coping mechanisms such as sense of humor, intellectualism, and denial to deal with stress.
4. Plan and execute tasks.
5. Choose to engage in higher cortical functions such as language.
6. Decision making/making judgements.

The frontal lobes require a lot of energy and may activate any area of the brain. It is not hard to see how sleep deprivation could affect frontal lobe function. Remember, sleep produces the "gas" or neurotransmitters needed for normal functions. If you run out of gas then you will have limited frontal lobe functioning (i.e., it is hard to function or the patient may complain of "brain fog").

Illness that are affected by sleep:

1. Sleep deprivation—induction of mania in bipolar patient
2. Sleep deprivation—induce migraines
3. Sleep deprivation—induce or promote seizures
4. REM sleep induction of panic attacks (Panic activates cortex, patient awakens in fear and panic and cannot go back to sleep)
5. Others such as immune disorders (low resistance to infections)

Examining **The Williams Brain Model for Sleep,** there are three elements for getting to sleep.
   1. Deactivation of cortex.
   2. Secretion of melatonin.
   3. Pull to sleep.

Figure 1-5: The Williams Brain Model

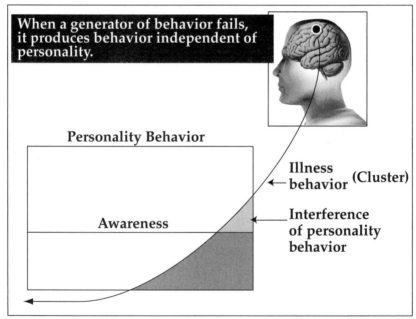

If there is a problem with one of the three steps in getting to sleep, the patient will complain of insomnia. If the patient complains of daytime tiredness or a tendency to sleep too much, then the problem lies within the sleep center. When the sleep center is unable to fill up the neurotransmitter gas tank during sleep, then daytime hypersomnolance follows. There may be a mechanism that blocks the sleep center's ability to fill up the neurotransmitter gas tank or there may be an inherent deficit in the sleep center that decreases the sleep center's ability to provide restorative sleep. In the case of sleep center problems, the patient does not have trouble getting to sleep. Because the patient is unable to pay back his sleep debt, he feels sleepy during the day (i.e., falls asleep easily). The patient is miserable trying to function because he feels tired and constantly is fighting the pull to go to sleep. In this clinic setting, we describe the problem as daytime hypersomnolance. Daytime hypersomnolance is related to the sleep center's inability to provide restorative sleep. Because the patient does not perceive a sleep problem, he/she may only complain of daytime sleeping.

In summary, we have two major subjective complaints related to sleep problems. One subjective complaint is related to insomnia or inability to get or stay asleep. The other involves daytime sleepiness (hypersomnolance) which is the inability to provide restorative sleep.

The following charts give information about sleep disorders interfering with functioning.

- Danger of drowsy driving
- Impact on daily activity

After review of the charts, it is obvious that sleep has a dramatic effect on our lives.

Figure 1-6: The danger of drowsy driving

According to the National Highway Traffic Safety Administration, thousands of vehicular crashes and injuries each year are attributed to sleepy, fatigued drivers.

Each year, drowsy driving causes…

Vehicular crashes	56,000
Nonfatal injuries	40,000
Fatalities	1,550

Adapted from: NCSDR/NHTSA Expert Panel on Driver Fatigue and Sleepiness. Drowsy driving and automobiles crashes (National Highway Traffic Safety Administration web site). Available at: *http://www.nhtsa.dot.gov/people/perform/human/Drowsy.html. Accessed February 22, 2000.*

Figure 1-7: Insomnia's impact on daily activities

A recent study of 261 individuals with insomnia and 101 people without sleep disorders showed that insomnia can have a substantial impact on everyday activities, including absences from work.

	Insomnia Patients	Healthy Controls
Days absent from work per month	1.32	0.13
Hours per day spent reading	1.91	2.36
Hours per day spent watching television	3.26	2.46

Source: Zammit GK, Weiner J, Damato N, et al. Quality of life in people with insomnia. *Sleep.* 1999;22(suppl 2):S379-S385.

The prevalence of insomnia in the United States ranges from 17.4 to 37.8 percent.[5] Daytime somnolance ranges from 4 to 12 percent.[6] Children are also affected.[7]

---

[1] Dr. Robert A. Williams' formulation for establishing biological stability of the brain.

[2,3] Breslau et al. *Biol Psychiatry.* 1996;39:411.

[4] Pg. 1140, *Principals and Practice of Sleep Medicine* Third Edition, Kryger, Roth and Dement.

[5] Klink ME, Quan SF, Icaltenborn WT, Lebowitz MR, Risk factors associated with complaints of insomnia in a general white population. *Arch Intern Med.* 1992:152:1634–1637.

[6] Roth T, Roehrs TA, Carkadon MA, Dement WC, Daytime sleepiness and alertness. In: Kryger MH, Roth T, Dement WC. Eds, *Principles & Practice of Sleep Medicine.* 2nd ed. Philadelphia PA; WB Saunders, 1994:40–41.

[7] Camhi SL, Morgan WJ, Pernisco N, Quan SF. Factors affecting sleep disturbances in children and adolescents. *Sleep Med.* 2000;1:117–123.

Summary of Introduction to *Brain Basics: Sleep*

1. Sleep is a necessary function for normal brain functioning and life.
2. Sleep is a unique altered state for the purpose of filling up the neurotransmitter gas tank and paying back energy debts.
3. The consequences of sleep dysfunction can affect all brain and bodily functions.
4. Sleep disorders are neurological or medical disorders that affect the brain.
5. Difficulty in getting or staying asleep usually results in the complaint of "insomnia."
6. Difficulty in getting restorative sleep usually results in the complaint of "daytime sleepiness."
7. There are three steps to get to sleep.
    a. Deactivate the cortex.
    b. Secrete the melatonin key.
    c. Pull to sleep based on sleep debt.
8. Restorative sleep is determined by the subjective sense that one is energetic and fully functional during the day (i.e., restored). Does the person have a full tank of gas to run his brain engine during the day?
9. Sleep disorders cause brain disorders, induce inherent brain disorders and adversely affect our functioning.
10. Sleep is an important parameter in determining biological stability in the psychiatric patient.
11. Lack of sleep contributes to industrial and automobile accidents.

Chapter 2

What is Sleep?

Stages of Sleep
Defining Normal Sleep

"All men whilst they are awake are in one common world:
but each of Them, when he is asleep, is in a world of his own."

PLUTARCH 46–120

"Frontal lobe awareness and control is our connection to the outer world.
Sleep involves transferring control from the frontal lobes to the sleep center."

ROBERT A. WILLIAMS, M.D.

Sleep is an altered brain state that usually occurs at night, for restorative purposes. The metabolic demands or energy needs of the brain in the awake state are too great to sustain brain activity for 24 hours. The brain needs a break (sleep) to restore its energy and neurotransmitter needs.

The energy requirements for nerve cells during awake states exceed what the brain can produce. Energy requirements include energy needs for changing nervous system structure as in memory consolidation. Brain cells require neurotransmitters for communication between cells and coordinating brain activity. The demands for producing neurotransmitters and neuroreceptors during the awake state exceed what a brain cell can provide. The brain cell acquires an energy and neurotransmitter/neuroreceptor debt during the awake state that is paid back during the sleep state (i.e., restoration). Thusly, sleep is an altered brain state that usually occurs at night for the purpose of restoring the brain cells back to a positive metabolic state (i.e., pay back the daytime debt) that allows for normal daytime functioning.

The brain is an information processing machine that has very high energy requirements. The brain is the primary organ system of the body (e.g., the organ system of existence). All other organ systems of the body have one primary function and that is to support the brain.

The heart pumps nutrients and oxygen to the brain; the gastrointestinal tract absorbs nutrients for the brain; the lungs absorb oxygen for the brain; the bones and muscles give the brain mobility; skin provides protection and an internal environment for the brain; and the kidneys provide an internal electrolyte environment for nervous system functions.

The brain is a very demanding organ system. The metabolic demands of all the organs and the brain are too great to sustain for 24 hours. During sleep, two major changes occur:

1. The metabolism of the other organ systems decreases. For example there is decrease of body functions and cortisol levels in the body that result in a decrease in overall metabolism. When overall metabolism decreases, energy can be shunted to the brain.
2. The brain switches from creating a metabolic debt to creating a neurotransmitter and metabolic reserve for awake use. Normal or awake brain function is turned off, so brain cells can be restored.

Thusly, the brain is a two-cycle machine, much like the heart. During the diastolic phase of the heart, the heart fills up with blood, in the systolic phase of the heart, the heart pumps out blood to provide nutrients to cells of the body. In the sleep phase, the brain fills up with neurotransmitter gas. During the awake phase, the brain discharges the neurotransmitter gas and energy to produce human behavior.

Note that the blood vessels in the brain respond to the metabolic needs by changing blood flow. When the metabolic needs of one part of the brain increase, the blood vessels to that part of the brain dilate and increase blood flow. It is this observation that allows scientists to measure metabolic rates of the brain by measuring blood flow.

The brain cells try to minimize the daytime metabolic debt by being efficient. For example, neurotransmitters are recycled into the brain cells for reuse. By reusing neurotransmitters the neurotransmitter reserve that is created the night before lasts longer.

Re-uptake mechanisms involve brain cells "pumping" the neurotransmitters back into the brain cell after the neurotransmitter has been discharged and utilized. It is much like a recycling process, as in recycling aluminum cans for reuse.

Re-uptake mechanisms have a modulating (modulation means control, so that thinking and movement can be orchestrated to provide adaptable behavior) function in addition to a reuse function. Biologically, a balance between the amount of neurotransmitters and the number of receptors is maintained. Re-uptake mechanisms (i.e., removal of neurotransmitters) help maintain that balance between neurotransmitter load and neurore-ceptor density.

The purpose of measuring sleep is to understand normal sleep mechanisms and how sleep can be disrupted. The patient's subjective sense of being restored, feeling well and functioning well is the bottom line in determining whether sleep is normal or abnormal (not the direct measuring of sleep). The average length of a full night's sleep is 8 hours or 480 minutes. Sleep consists of 90- to 100-minute cycles or about 5 cycles per night. Stage 1 and 2 sleep (or light sleep) followed by Stage 3 and 4 sleep (or deep sleep) followed by REM sleep (Rapid Eye Movement or dream sleep). The electrical activity of the brain, as measured by the electrocephalogram (EEG), is the major determinate of the stages of sleep (see Figure 2-2). An example is the EEG measurement of deep or slow wave sleep.[1]

As mentioned in ***Brain Basics***®, there are four kinds of behavior. Behavior is anything that reflects brain activity. The different kinds of behavior are: (1) overt; (2) electrical and magnetic; (3) neuroendocrine; and (4) metabolic. (Note that blood flow can be an indirect measure of metabolic behavior.)

Measuring the electrical behavior of the brain is how we measure stages of sleep. Electrical activity of the brain is measured by the EEG. The electrical activity of the brain is a continuous electrical discharge that is recorded as waves. The loss of brain waves is one criteria in determining brain death. The waves are measured by location on the head, size of wave and frequency (number of cycles per second). Usually our awake waves are 8 to 12 cycles per second (alpha waves) or faster. When we are awake our frontal lobes have low voltage fast activity indicating cortical activation. When we are in deep sleep, the cortex has high voltage slow waves indicating cortical deactivation and control by the sleep center deep in the brain. The sleep center synchronizes the activity of the cortical brain cells to produce high voltage slow waves. The stages of sleep are based on the electrical pattern seen on the EEG. The following figure is a list of brain wave frequencies.

Figure 2-1: Brain Wave Frequencies

alpha waves	8–12 cycles/sec—awake pattern	
beta waves (fast)	25–35 cycles/sec—awake pattern	Based on the brain wave pattern, stages of sleep are determined.
Delta waves (slow)	2–5 cycles/sec—seen in Stage 3 and 4 sleep (slow wave sleep)	
Theta	3–7 cycles/sec—seen in Stage 1 and Stage 2 sleep	

K complexes and spindles are complex waves seen in Stage 2 sleep

Sleep is the only normal behavior in which defined states are measured by the EEG. Even though defined states are defined by the EEG, it is the subjective (how one feels) and the functional aspects of one's life that determines the normalcy of sleep.

Figure 2-2: Brain Wave Patterns and Stages of Sleep

	EEG Characteristics (brain waves)
Stage 1 & 2 (*light sleep*)	Break up of awake brain waves and resting alpha rhythms awake resting brain waves and production of K complexes (complex rhythm that is specific for Stage 2 sleep). Less than 20 percent of the record is slow wave activity.
Stage 3 & 4 (*deep sleep*)	Slow wave sleep. On any given EEG page, if the percent of slow waves exceeds 50 percent, then it is Stage 4 sleep. If it is less than 50 percent and greater than 20 percent, then it is Stage 3 sleep. Slow wave sleep is therefore > 20 percent of slow waves.
Rapid Eye Movement (*REM*)	Slow wave sleep is replaced by low voltage fast activity that is similar to the awake EEG (i.e., activation of the cortex).

There are many physiological changes that occur during the different stages of sleep. The following is a chart describing a few of the clinically significant physiological changes.

Figure 2-3: Physiological Changes and Stages of Sleep

	Autonomic Breathing	Muscle Tone	Autonomic Heart Rate	Spinal Reflexes* (ability to stand)	Body Temperature
Light Sleep	Normal	Normal	Normal	None	Normal
Deep Sleep	Slower	Decreased (partial paralysis)	Slower	None	Cooler
REM	Faster	Paralysis	Increased	None	Body is not temperature regulated (i.e., assumes environmental temperature)

*You cannot stand and be asleep. If you go to sleep standing you will fall down because of loss of spinal cord reflexes. Spinal cord reflexes create muscle tone in a way that allows us to stand up without a conscious effort.

Superimposed on the immediate physiological changes that occur during sleep are the diurnal physiological changes. At night around 11 P.M. our cortisol levels decrease and our body temperature decreases. Presumably, the lower cortisol and lower body temperature reflect a lower overall metabolic rate for the entire body. The lower overall metabolic rate allows metabolic resources to be redirected to the brain for the restoration of the brain.

The bottom line in determining if a person has normal sleep is whether or not a person feels well and functions well during the awake state. If a person feels energetic, mood is stable and does not feel tired or sleepy, the prior night's sleep was restorative.

As mentioned, sleep consolidates memory. Therefore, there is a close relationship between sleep and memory. Memory begins as a biochemical entity. With sleep, memory is translated into a structural form (i.e., consolidated).

When the neurotransmitters are delivered to the nerve terminal during REM sleep, overflow occurs. The overflow causes dreams. Strangely enough, the brain wave pattern of the cortex during dreams appears like the awake pattern of the cortex. Awake and REM sleep brain wave patterns involve low voltage, fast (high frequency) brain waves. The person dreaming is paralyzed, so there is no motor response (movement) to dreaming. Depending on the individual and the state of memory, dreams can take on a large variety of content-of-life issues. The following is a list of examples:

1. A patient stated his parents taught him to always be insecure about work and to never be satisfied with his work accomplishments. The patient, in spite of being successful, had continuous dreams about working harder that were exhausting and unpleasant. I counseled the patient that he had a long history of childhood memories that were activated by his neurotransmitter overflow during dreaming. I suggested meditation at bedtime of positive thoughts to substitute for the negative childhood experience. With time and effort, he was able to change his dream content.

   Most of us automatically do a meditation process and have positive dreams. Some persons need to be proactive to have pleasant dreams.

2. Instinctive needs are reflected in dreams. They can be as basic as hunger (dreaming about eating), need to urinate or sexual.

3. Creative processes are reflected in dreams. Creative persons meditate and have deep reflective thoughts that can be activated during dream states.

   Dreams are the bystander of information in memory that may be captured by the overflow of neurotransmitters during REM sleep.

4. Illness behavior can be reflected in dreams. For instance, suicidal thoughts related to depression can be reflected in dreams.

   It is thought that dreams activate existing memories, so that any memories occurring during sleep can be remembered during the awake state. For the most part, dreaming does not provide any unique capacity to stimulate memory. For instance, if a patient has dreams of suicide, related to depression, the patient is always aware of suicidal thoughts during the awake state.

   Defense mechanisms or coping mechanisms may distort or block a person's memory of an event. Analysts feel that interpretation of certain dreams in the setting of absent awake defense mechanisms helps patients understand and "work through" psychological traumas or, perhaps in some cases, even identify the traumas.

Restorative enzymes convert amino acids to neurotransmitters such as dopamine and seratonin. (Amino acids are unique molecules that are the building blocks of proteins. Proteins are digested and broken down into amino acids that are absorbed into the blood stream and ultimately transported to the brain. Dopamine and seratonin are molecules that are utilized by brain cells to communicate between brain cells.) Genetically, the amount and efficiency of restorative enzymes vary, thus the amount of sleep one needs varies. The average amount of sleep is 8 hours, some persons need more than 8 hours depending on how efficiently restorative enzymes work.

If a person does not get enough sleep to fill up his/her neurotransmitter gas tank, they will develop a sleep debt. For instance, a college student who needs 8 hours of sleep a night will develop a sleep debt of one hour per night if he/she gets only 7 hours of sleep per night. Then, during the weekend he/she will pay back the debt by sleeping longer on Saturday and Sunday.

There are neurological changes that occur during sleep.

Figure 2-4: Neurological Phenomena Associated with Sleep

Awake Awareness	a sense of being awake or not asleep.
Sleep Awareness	vague sense of being asleep. Less interaction with environmental stimuli.
Alerting Mechanism	multiple mechanisms can occur that activate the cortex for awake functioning. All alerting mechanisms are turned off during sleep.
Spinal Reflexes	antigravity spinal reflexes are lost in all stages of sleep—you *cannot* stand up while sleeping.
Muscle Tone	muscle tone is decreased in Stage 3 and 4 sleep and all muscle tone is lost in REM sleep. Stage 1 and Stage 2 sleep have the most muscle tone seen during sleep.

Spinal reflexes are antigravity spinal reflexes. Muscle tone without spinal reflexes is the activation of the muscle at rest which resists movement, (that is not directly antigravity).

Memory function: active memory formulation as a result of interaction with the environment is reduced or lost during sleep. Memory recovery during sleep may reflect underlying attitudes. Past content-of-life issues may be reflected in dreams. Persons with Post-Traumatic Stress Disorder may awaken during a dream that reflects his/her trauma.

Sleep status during awake states reflects:
- enough sleep—a sense of being restored
- length of sleep—a sense of having slept enough
- sense of having been asleep

There is a melatonin "gas tank" that usually takes seventeen hours to fill. The melatonin gas tank is filled during the day when a person is awake. After seventeen hours, the overflow stimulates the release of eight hours of melatonin (i.e., melatonin reaches threshold levels that allow darkness to stimulate the release of melatonin, thus there is an intrinsic twenty-five hour sleep/wake cycle). When the melatonin "tank" is near full, darkness stimulates its release thus allowing for entrainment (i.e., synchronizing sleep with night and day). Entrainment is coordinating sleep with darkness overnight. While we are filling up on melatonin, we use up our neurotransmitter gas during the day. During the night while we are using the melatonin gas, we fill up our neurotransmitter tank.

Sleep involves getting to sleep and, once asleep, getting restorative sleep. Getting to sleep involves a three-step process:
1. Deactivation of the cortex.
2. Secretion of melatonin.
3. Pull to sleep.

Once a person is asleep, then there are three steps to restorative sleep.
1. Transport of amino acids (light sleep).
2. Synthesizing neurotransmitters (deep sleep).
3. Delivery of the neurotransmitters to the nerve terminal (REM sleep).

Getting to sleep involves accessing the sleep center and giving control to the sleep center. Once the sleep center is in control, then it is a matter of production and delivery of neurotransmitters and paying back energy debts that occurred during the day. One function that occurs during the day that requires high energy is memory. It is thought that depending on emotional states, memories are selectively consolidated during sleep (i.e., converted from a temporary biochemical form to a structural form). There are processes that can deactivate the cortex but do not activate restorative sleep. For example, alcohol overuse can deactivate the cortex, but poison the sleep center capacity to restore the brain. Alcoholics sleep a lot, but never get restful sleep.

The hypothalamus is a major structure of the limbic system that relates to homeostasis and motivational states that influence survival and reproduction. The hypothalamus is a system of nuclei (groups of brain cells) that measures the status of systems and provides awareness and motivation to maintain an external and internal environment for survival and reproductive purposes. There are many physical parameters that the hypothalamus measures such as osmolality, glucose levels, food requirements and many others. There is an area of the hypothalamus that measures adequacy of sleep or need for sleep. It is the neurotransmitter reserve and metabolic debt that are measured in the hypothalamus. If the hypothalamus gas tank reflects full, then presumably the entire brain tank is full. There is a rare condition in which the hypothalamus tank is defective and the patient has the subjective sense of not having had restorative sleep when in fact the brain is restored. Most of the time, the hypothalamic tank represents an accurate reflection of the entire status of the brain. This is similar to a gas tank gauge that is defective, showing empty when, indeed, the tank is full.

Figure 2-5: Williams Brain Model showing the three steps needed to get to sleep.

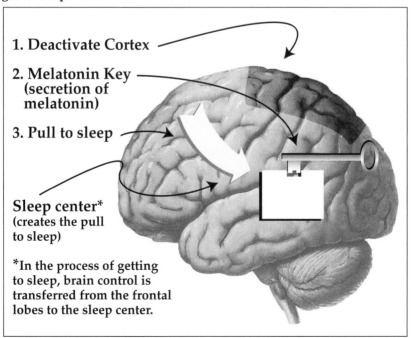

1. Deactivate Cortex

2. Melatonin Key
   (secretion of
   melatonin)

3. Pull to sleep

Sleep center*
(creates the pull
to sleep)

*In the process of getting
to sleep, brain control is
transferred from the frontal
lobes to the sleep center.

In summary, there are two common complaints associated with sleep disorders:
1. Insomnia, which is related to getting and staying asleep.
2. Daytime hypersomnalance, which is related to getting restorative sleep (tired with desire or tendency to go to sleep).

Executive function involves modulating other generators of behavior (i.e., orchestrating the different generators of behavior to be adaptable to content of life). If a person becomes aware of being tired, he can resist it willfully. Of course, any instinctual behavior such as appetite and sleep can be resisted but not without great effort. And, the instinctual behaviors are always obsessional (i.e. constant intrusive thoughts). One danger of inadequate sleep is falling asleep at an inappropriate time. If a person is driving and cannot sustain the resistance to sleep, disaster will follow.

Summary of what is sleep:
1. Sleep is an altered brain state for restorative purposes.
2. The purpose of sleep is to restore neurotransmitters and energy reserves. The brain engine (personality) runs on neurotransmitter gas and energy during the awake state.
3. The hypothalamus and brain stem (i.e., sleep center) control and measure sleep.
4. There are three steps needed to get to sleep and there are three steps needed to get restorative sleep.
5. The EEG measures the stages of sleep. Adequacy of sleep is a subjective assessment made on a person's sense of feeling awake during the day, feeling normal and functioning normally.

[1] *Principles and Practice of Sleep Medicine* by Kryger Roth Dement, WB Saunders Company©2000, pg. 20

SECTION 2

GETTING TO SLEEP (3 STEPS)

Chapter 3

Overview of What is Needed to Get to Sleep

"They say we sleep to let the demons out—to let the men go raving mad, our dreams and nightmares all our logic gone awry, the dark side of our reason. And when the daylight comes again…comes order with it."

AGNES (WIFE OF TOBIAS)

ACT III

"A DELICATE BALANCE"

BY EDWARD ALBEE (BORN 1928)

"We have little conscious control over sleep processes."

ROBERT A. WILLIAMS, M.D.

The process of evolution has created an advanced central nervous system (CNS) to facilitate survival and procreation in the human brain. The energy needed to sustain the CNS during active periods exceeded the biological energy capacity of living systems. The CNS evolved as a two-cycle machine. As CNS energy requirements increased, so did the efficiency needs of sleep. Efficiency is defined as restorative energy divided by total energy expended. The brain and body try to use minimal energy during sleep so that energy can be used as restorative energy. For example, a decrease in brain temperature decreases brain metabolism. Spinal reflexes are lost during sleep (i.e., one cannot stand up during sleep), thus the energy used to maintain spinal reflexes is conserved and can be used for restorative energy.

The sleep center has relative control over neurotransmitters that control the cortex of the brain and spinal cord. Note that as a person experiences sleep, there is progressive paralysis and decreased ability to be aroused. There is minimal interaction with the environment and no new memory formulation with the environment. Norepinephrine is turned off which causes paralysis. Dopamine is turned off which causes unconsciousness. Acytylcholine is turned off which causes active memory function to stop. Seratonin is turned off which causes a decrease in overall emotional arousal. Histamine which is specific to the sleep center and activates the frontal lobe executive center is turned off. In summary, the neurotransmitter systems that activate the cortex for daytime human behavior are turned off by the sleep center.

In order to define sleep, one might ask, "What is the state of being asleep?" Sleep is a brain state in which the sleep center of the brain is in control allowing for restorative sleep. Restorative sleep involves the following functions:

1. Consolidate memory.
2. Produce and deliver neurotransmitters to the nerve terminal for use the next day.
3. Pay back energy debt.

Getting to sleep is a three-step process. The first is to shut down the cortex. The second is to secrete melatonin, the key that opens the sleep center door. The third is a pull to sleep from the sleep center.

The cortex is a specialized part of the brain located on the surface of the brain. The cortex is a vital part of the brain that contains awareness, capacity to plan and execute tasks and higher cortical functioning such as abstract thinking. The cortex has high energy and neurotransmitter demands. In order to pay back energy debts and to provide a neurotransmitter reserve, the cortex must be shut down during sleep (i.e., deactivate).

In order to devote as much energy as possible to restoring the brain, energy demands for the entire body are reduced during sleep. Our body temperature and cortisol secretion are reduced at night in order to decrease energy demands. During REM (rapid eye movement) sleep, the body becomes poikilothermic (i.e., there is no temperature regulation or the body tends to assume the environmental temperature). This further decreases body energy demands and allows for the final phase of brain restoration during REM sleep.

Basically, any process that counters the usual processes of sleep may disturb sleep. For example, if a person exercises at night metabolism and

Figure 3-1: Diagram showing the physical requirements for getting to sleep.

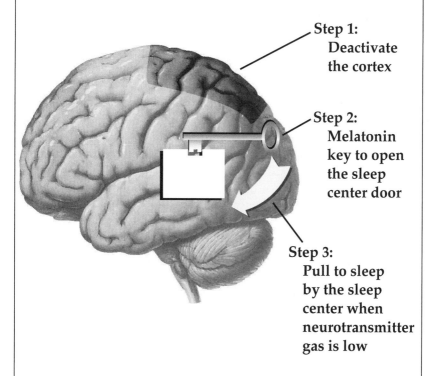

Williams Brain Model

Three Steps To Get To Sleep

Sleep is a process that creates neurotransmitter gas and energy that runs the brain engine the next day.

There are three steps needed to get to sleep.

Step 1:
   Deactivate
   the cortex

Step 2:
   Melatonin
   key to open
   the sleep
   center door

Step 3:
   Pull to sleep
   by the sleep
   center when
   neurotransmitter
   gas is low

When a patient is unable to get to sleep he will complain of "insomnia."

body temperatures go up. This counters the tendency of lowering the body temperature and metabolism during sleep. Thus, exercise at night may disturb sleep onset. One sleep hygiene recommendation is to exercise early in the day to avoid sleep disturbance. Sleep hygiene is advice on how to create an environment that facilitates sleep. The effect of countering the usual processes of sleep decreases the pull of the sleep center and decreases the sleep center's capacity to turn off the cortex.

Another example of how countering normal sleep onset physiology can disturb sleep is emotional upset. For instance, if a wife and husband have an argument. Anger and/or rage can activate the cortex and increase cortisol levels in the body. Thus, after a heated argument, a person may find it difficult to get to sleep.

The basic question is "What mechanisms can potentially interfere with cortical deactivation?" There are eight basic mechanisms that can interfere with cortical deactivation.

1. External sensory stimulus. An example is loud noise.
2. Internal sensory stimulus. An example is gastric reflux causing pain or urge to urinate.
3. Internal instinctive stimulus. An example is hunger causing a person to awaken and want to eat.
4. Overactivated personality generators of behavior or illness behavior. An example is obsessive worry or activation of the reticular activating system (RAS) from a spousal argument.
5. Sleep generator may have a weak capacity to pull control to the sleep center or to reduce the RAS—overactivation (Primary insomnia).
6. Willfully countering the urge to sleep.
7. Drugs.
8. Conditioning (i.e., bad habits of sleep).

Heightening of any awareness modality may interfere with cortical deactivation. Within the frontal lobes, humans have a large and unique capacity for awareness. Awareness can involve time (past, present, future), environment, body, cognition (thinking), etc.

Any stimulation of *sensory awareness* can interrupt sleep. External sensory stimulation of the nervous system can involve heat, vibration, pain, sound (auditory), smell (olfaction) or taste (gustatory). Internal sensory stimulation of the nervous system can involve pain such as gastric reflux or colonic spasms. Internal stimulation of the nervous system can involve bladder

Figure 3-2: Impeding Cortical Deactivation

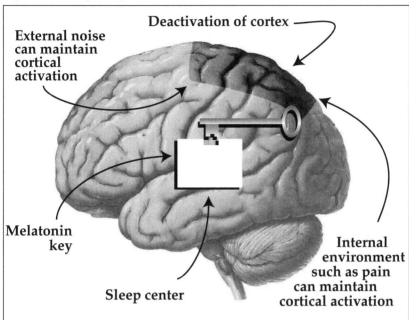

External Sources of Activation include any stimulation of the sensory system: heat, pain, vibration, sound, smell (olfaction) or taste (gustatory)

Internal Sources of Activation include instincts such as hunger or pain such as gastro-esophageal reflux (GERD)

contractions that can awaken a person to urinate. Instincts such as hunger pains can cause heightened awareness and awaken a person.

Internal stimulation of the cortex can occur from personality generators of behavior. For instance, a person may be under stress during the day. Stress may cause generalized anxiety disorder or obsessive worry and can cause insomnia (difficulty getting to sleep) or interrupted sleep (restless sleep). Fear may activate the reticular activating system making it difficult to go to sleep.

Another example of internal stimulation of the cortex is willfully countering the urge to sleep. An example is the person who, in spite of being tired, watches a late-night movie. The individual is required to get up and to go to work and thus becomes sleep deprived. Willfully countering the urge to sleep is a common mechanism in our culture to prevent cortical deactivation.

Sleep hygiene advice commonly suggests that people use their will to go to bed at the same time each night at a reasonable hour that will provide adequate sleep time (i.e., approximately eight hours).

Some persons have weak sleep generators of behavior that lead to chronic insomnia. Without a knowledge of sleep hygiene, these disorders can progress to severe forms causing disability. If the primary cause of insomnia is a weak sleep generator it is called primary insomnia.

Drugs can have a profound effect on sleep in three ways:
1. Direct effect on sleep.
2. Withdrawal effects on sleep.
3. Indirect effects on sleep.

One example of the direct effects on sleep is alcohol use to get to sleep, the so-called "night cap." Alcohol can cause sedation and help counter anxiety and obsessive worry. But, once a person is asleep, alcohol suppresses REM sleep and thus alcohol lessens restorative sleep. The patient will state, "I slept, but awoke unrested and tired."

Since alcohol is metabolized relatively quickly, alcohol withdrawal effects can interrupt sleep. As alcohol is metabolized (i.e., withdrawn from the body), the sedative (calming) effects are replaced by activating effects. The activating withdrawal effects of alcohol may even awaken the patient and even prompt further alcohol use.

Because alcohol has toxic effects on the brain, alcohol can indirectly affect sleep. Alcohol stimulates the release of dopamine and other neurotransmitters. If alcohol is used chronically, then neurotransmitter stores become depleted. The depletion of neurotransmitter stores can lead to depression. In extreme cases, heavy chronic use of alcohol can cause confusion, hallucinations and agitation (i.e., delirium). The brain consequences of depression and delirium include insomnia. Thus, alcohol effects sleep directly and indirectly. To summarize, alcohol use is not good for sleep.

For some patients there is a window of opportunity to get to sleep. Sleep is an instinct and subject to limbic system reward and punishment. The amount of limbic system punishment (angst) varies with the individual. For example some people become very irritable if they do not eat a meal on time. Others become very anxious even with a small loss in the stock market (gathering instinct). For patients with strong limbic system response to lack of sleep, a window of opportunity to get to sleep can be created.

In the evening when neurotransmitter gas levels are low, one experiences tiredness. The tiredness is the sleep center pull to go to sleep. The sleep center turns off activation of the frontal lobe creating awareness of being tired.

At a certain point, limbic system activation will occur if the person does not go to sleep. If the limbic system activation is high, it may counter the sleep center's pull to go to sleep. The time between the beginning of the sleep center pull to go to sleep and the limbic system's reaction to not going to sleep is the window of opportunity to get to sleep. If a patient goes to sleep too early there is not enough pull from the sleep. If a patient goes to sleep too late there is too much limbic system activation to get to sleep.

Figure 3-3: Window of Opportunity to Get to Sleep

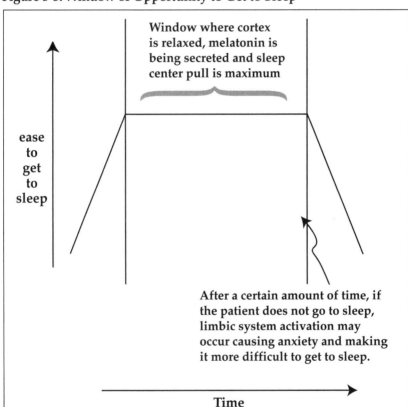

The basic strategy of sleep hygiene is to minimize activation of the nervous system in order to enhance deactivation of the cortex and to avoid negative conditioning of sleep (negative attitude towards sleep).

There can be emotional responses that occur when we unsuccessfully try to go to sleep. Sleep is an essential part of survival in life (i.e., an instinct). The purpose of the limbic system (i.e., emotion) is to provide motivations to carry out instinctive drives. If an instinct is successfully carried out, the limbic system rewards us with dopamine release, and we have a natural high. If an instinct is not satisfied, then the limbic system punishes us with anxiety and depression. The limbic system provides positive reinforcement with success and negative reinforcement with failure. When we fail to go to sleep, there is a profound negative emotional response from the limbic system. Thus, if a person can't get go sleep within twenty minutes, it is recommended to get up and to focus on another activity. The association between the negative emotions of not being able to go to sleep and being in bed can be so great that the person can't sleep from this mechanism alone. This is called psycho-physiological response.

The puzzling thing about psycho-physiological response is that even if you correct the problem that caused the initial insomnia, the psycho-physiological response (or the negative emotion about sleep) may continue and cause insomnia in itself. In other words, the stimulus that creates insomnia creates a negative conditioning towards sleep.

The same principle applies to positive associations with sleep. If a person is always watching television when they go to sleep, they may not be able to go to sleep without the television. Or, if a person takes a sleeping pill in association with sleep, then the person may not be able to get to sleep without a sleeping pill. Sleep hygiene includes a caution about the powerful instinctive emotional responses related to sleep and the ease of creating negative associations with sleep or maladaptive positive associations with sleep.

Anything that is associated with powerful instincts such as sleep are quickly reinforced, either positively or negatively.

Any environmental threat, real or imagined, will prevent the cortex from being deactivated. One can see this as an evolutionary protective mechanism. If a person is under a threat, going to sleep would be a great disadvantage. The activation of the cortex provided by the threat will maintain wakefullness and prevent inappropriate sleep.

Since deactivation of the cortex is just one of three requirements to get to sleep, deactivation of the cortex alone will not be sufficient for restorative sleep. When a patient is under anesthesia, the patient uniquely is disconnected from pain, but not necessarily getting restorative sleep. Note that normal sleep will not disconnect pain awareness. Thus, deactivation of the cortex alone may give the appearance of sleep, but does not necessarily mean a person is "sleeping."

The second physical requirement needed to get to sleep is melatonin secretion. Melatonin is the key that opens up the sleep center door to allow sleep.

Melatonin secretion is inhibited by light, or conversely, darkness tends to encourage the release of melatonin. The purpose of melatonin secretion is to entrain (coordinate) sleep with nighttime.

When melatonin secretion is delayed from desired sleep time, it may cause a delay in sleep, or a delayed sleep syndrome. When melatonin secretion is released earlier than desired sleep time, it may cause earlier sleep or advanced sleep phase syndrome. More information about melatonin secretion and disorders of melatonin secretion will be supplied in another chapter.

The third physical requirement for sleep is the pull to sleep. During the day when the brain is active, energy and neurotransmitter requirements exceed what the brain can maintain. After a full day of activity, the brain runs low on neurotransmitter and energy gas (e.g., creates an energy debt). Because the brain restores neurotransmitters and energy reserves during sleep, the phenomena of being tired at night causes the pull to sleep. When the sleep debt is "paid off" after a good night's sleep, then the pull to sleep resolves.

Nature designed the brain engine to run during the day and designed sleep in order to fill up the neurotransmitter gas tank at night.

Nature designed the brain to operate on a two-cycle process. The first cycle, sleep at night, is for the purpose of filling up the neurotransmitter gas tank. The second cycle, awake during the day, is to produce behavior for survival and reproductive purposes. In other words, sleep provides the gas for the brain engine to run the next day.

When the sleep center is low on neurotransmitter gas, the sleep center does three things to prepare for sleep.

1. Decreases RAS (reticular activating system) activity to allow for cortical deactivations. The RAS activates the cortex and decreases the secretion of histamine which also activates the cortex.
2. Pulls control from the cortex to the sleep center.
3. Decreases energy demands by the body by decreasing cortisol, decreasing body temperature, decreasing motor activity, eliminating spinal reflexes and decreasing motor tone, among others.

Conceptually, sleep hygiene supports physiological mechanisms that encourage cortical deactivation and reinforce sleep center physiology.

Sleep hygiene (advice that facilitates sleep) involves enhancing normal sleep mechanisms and avoiding things that can disrupt sleep.

Factors that enhance normal sleep mechanisms can include:
1. Cool room.
2. Low metabolic rate (don't exercise late in the day).
3. Sleep at the same time to enhance sleep cycle or rhythm. The more regular the sleep rhythm, the more regular sleep is.

4. Avoid naps. If a person fills up his neurotransmitter gas tank too much, there will be less "pull" by the sleep center to go to sleep.

Avoid things that can disrupt sleep by cortical activation such as:
1. Avoid noise that may prevent deactivation of the cortex.
2. Avoid emotional stimulation. Activation of the reticular activating system can prevent deactivation of the cortex.
3. Avoid drugs that stimulate the cortex and prevent cortical deactivation such as caffeine or nicotine.
4. Avoid negative or maladaptive positive conditioning of sleep.

Sleep Rules

1. *Sleep Hygiene*—reinforce deactivation of cortex and reinforce sleep physiology.
2. *Meditation*—To disconnect generators of behavior that disrupt sleep (internal brain generators such as worry).
3. Avoid *drugs* that disrupt sleep.
4. Avoid *conditioning*—negative or maladaptive positive conditioning.

In summary, there are three physical requirements needed to get to sleep:
1. Deactivation of the cortex of the brain.
2. Melatonin secretion.
3. Pull to sleep.

Sleep hygiene is advice on how to deactivate the cortex and facilitate sleep:
1. Reinforce normal physiological mechanisms for sleep, such as avoiding exercise at night that raises body temperature.
2. Avoid things that interrupt sleep, such as noise.
3. Avoid associations with sleep that are maladaptive, such as staying in bed longer than twenty minutes when you can't sleep.
4. Avoid drugs that interrupt sleep, such as caffeine.
5. Relax and meditate in an attempt to disconnect personality generators of behavior, such as obsessive worry.

Sleep problems are common. Some persons have very strong sleep generators and never have problems with sleep. Other persons have normal sleep generators of behavior and will, on occasion, have problems with sleep. Still others have weak sleep generators of behavior and struggle with sleep on a constant basis.

Sleep hygiene is important to understand for two reasons:

1. Proper sleep hygiene usually helps with sleep and helps individuals avoid reliance on over-the-counter drugs and avoid sleep deprivation or a sleep debt.

2. Facilitated use of sleep hygiene helps people avoid maladaptive associations with sleep that can be worse than the original cause of insomnia.

The following three chapters will examine each of the three steps to get to sleep.

Chapter 4

Cortical Deactivation (Step 1)

"Sleep is the time to restore the machine of existence."

ROBERT A. WILLIAMS, M.D.

*"The purpose of sleep is to fill up the neurotransmitter and energy
gas tank to run the brain engine during the day."*

ROBERT A. WILLIAMS, M.D.

C ortical deactivation is one of the three steps to get to sleep. The three
steps are: (1) cortical deactivation; (2) melatonin secretion and (3) pull
to sleep.

Cortical activation/deactivation mechanisms are complex. There are
two mechanisms that predominate: (1) activation/deactivation of the
reticular activating system (RAS) and (2) pull to the sleep center.

There are two main brain states.

The activation of the reticular activating system (RAS) activates the cortex in the brain. Activation of the cortex of the brain maintains wakefulness
and frontal lobe executive function control. Other activating systems include the release of histamine and the release of acetylcholine. The sleep
center turns off all cortical activating systems in the process of getting to
sleep. Uniquely, the sleep center releases histamine in the process of maintaining wakefulness.

When the brain is in the *awake* state, the frontal lobes are in control, neurotransmitter and energy reserves are high, the RAS is activated and there
is no pull to go to sleep from the sleep center.

When the brain is in the *sleep* state, the sleep center is in control, neurotransmitter and energy reserves are low, the RAS is deactivated and there

is a strong pull from the sleep center. The sleep center creates its pull to sleep by turning off histamine release (another activating system) and signaling the limbic system to motivate the frontal lobes to initiate sleep (i.e., create dysphoria if sleep is not achieved).

Figure 4-1: Mechanisms for Awake and Sleep States

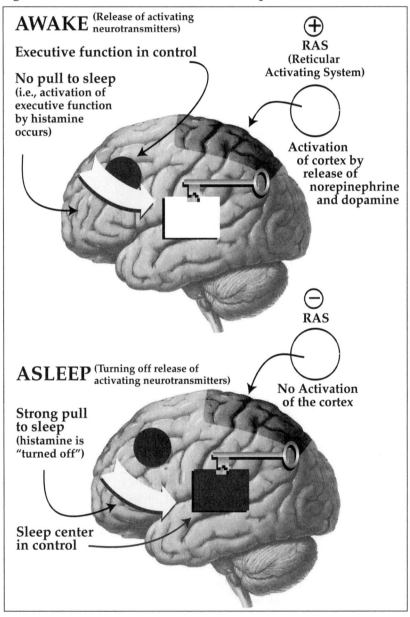

There are override mechanisms to cortical deactivation that arose through evolution. The override mechanisms are protective so that an organism can be awake for emergencies. Fear or pain are examples of cortical input that can override the normal sleep cycle and keep the organism awake.

As with all generators of the brain, there are individual differences in the strength of a given generator of behavior. Strong sleep generators will shut down the RAS and have strong pull from the frontal cortex to the sleep center. Persons with strong sleep generators will have a high capacity for sleep and minor emotional problems will not prevent cortical deactivation or sleep.

On the other hand, some persons have a weak sleep generator. The clinical syndrome, insomnia, due to a weak sleep generator relative to cortical activation is called primary insomnia. Primary insomnia is primary in that the cause is inherent to the sleep generator as opposed to being secondary to an external cause such as seizures occurring during sleep.

A weak sleep generator can be weak in relationship to the two requirements for sleep.

1. Weak in getting or staying asleep, which is related to cortical deactivation (primary insomnia).
2. Weak in providing restorative sleep (i.e., filling up the neurotransmitter tank [primary hypersomnia]).

It is thought that a weak sleep generator as applied to getting to sleep involves the balance of the RAS (activation) and the pull to sleep. If the deactivation of the RAS is incomplete, the patient will have trouble getting to sleep. Or, if the pull to sleep is weak compared to the activation of the RAS, the patient will have trouble getting to sleep. If both the RAS is overactive, and the pull to sleep is weak, the patient will probably have chronic, severe insomnia.

The brain is a two-cycle machine based on the two brain states. Cycle 1 is the sleep state where initially the energy and neurotransmitter reserves are low. During sleep, energy and neurotransmitter reserves are restored. Cycle 2 is the awake state where initially the neurotransmitter levels are high. The neurotransmitter gas is utilized during the awake state to produce human behavior.

Other biological systems are also two-cycle machines. For instance, the heart functions with two cycles. The diastolic cycle of heart function involves filling up the ventricles with blood. Similarly, the brain fills up with neurotransmitter gas. The systolic cycle of heart function involves pumping nutrients and oxygen to cells in the body. Similarly, the discharge of neurotransmitters during the awake state and the utilization of energy reserves creates human behavior.

It is important to note that all brain disorders have psychological consequences. For instance, patients with chronic illnesses develop obsessive worry about getting well, and when they get well, they obsessively worry about getting sick. Likewise, patients with sleep disorders develop psychological consequences. In Chapter 3, I discuss psycho-physiological sleep disturbances. "Pyscho" refers to the psychological attitude of the patient and physiological refers to the physiological consequences of negative attitudes. For instance, patients who go to bed and stay in bed despite the inability to sleep, develop a very negative attitude about sleep. The negative attitude can in itself activate the cortex and prevent sleep, hence the term psycho-physiological. A common cause of inability to deactivate the cortex is psycho-physiological. Any problem that can prevent sleep onset can cause psycho-physiological sleep disturbances. Thus, the sources of psycho-physiological problems are many, which makes psycho-physiological problems a common cause of inability to deactivate the cortex.

The following are examples of common problems involved with cortical deactivation:

Clinical Example 1 – *Generalized Anxiety Disorder* and insomnia

Clinical Example 2 – Insomnia due to *environmental noise*

Clinical Example 3 – Insomnia due to *caffeine use*

Clinical Example 4 – *Primary* insomnia

Clinical Example 5 – Insomnia due to *dyspepsia*

The following table summarizes causes of insomnia related to deactivation of the cortex. Note, in one case, if the cortex is overactivated, it will offset the pull to sleep. In the other case, if the pull to sleep is disrupted then resultant cortical activation can predominate.

Figure 4-2:

CAUSES OF INSOMNIA RELATED TO DEACTIVATION OF CORTEX
BALANCE BETWEEN ACTIVATION OF THE CORTEX AND DEACTIVATION

Activate Cortex	Interrupt Sleep Center Pull
Environmental (sleep hygiene) • Noise • Threat *Intrinsic Generator of Behavior (meditation)* • Obsessive worry • Anxiety *Medication* • Caffeine (discontinue use) *Negative Attitude Towards Sleep (meditation)* • Conditioned negative thoughts about sleep *Reticular Activation System (RAS) Overactivation (absolute or relative)* • Intrinsic activation of cortex that overrides sleep center pull to go to sleep or pull to sleep is weak (meditation) (relates to primary insomnia)	Weak intrinsic capacity to pull or deactivate the cortex. *Drugs* that interrupt sleep center activity—i.e., decrease sleep efficiency such as SSRIs. *Sleep-related illnesses* that interrupt sleep center activity such as Obstructive Sleep Apnea (OSA), Restless Leg Syndrome and Periodic Limb Movements of Sleep. *Medical illnesses* that interrupt sleep center activity such as Chronic Fatigue Syndrome, delirium and others. *Psychological illnesses* such as Post Trauma Stress Disorder—example, patient awakens with a terrifying dream. *Neurological illnesses* such as multiple seizures during sleep may interrupt sleep. *Psychiatric illnesses* such as depression can cause interrupted sleep.

Clinical Example 1: RAS Activation that Prevents Cortical Deactivation (clinical example involving deactivation of the cortex)

A 47-year-old male, married with two children, worked for an aerospace corporation as an engineer. The patient presented with difficulty going to sleep (i.e., insomnia for six months). The patient's problems began when his aerospace company began laying off employees. The patient had a past history of Generalized Anxiety Disorder (GAD) when faced with stress as noted in his college years. The patient satisfied the DSM IV criteria for GAD[1].

Diagnostic criteria for 300.02 Generalized Anxiety Disorder

A. Excessive anxiety and worry (apprehensive expectation), occurring for more days than not for at least 6 months, about a number of events or activities (such as work or school performance).

B. The person finds it difficult to control the worry.

C. The anxiety and worry are associated with three (or more) of the following six symptoms (with at least some symptoms present for more days than not for the past 6 months). Note: Only one item is required in children.
   (1) Restlessness or feeling keyed up or on edge
   (2) Being easily fatigued
   (3) Difficulty concentrating or mind going blank
   (4) Irritability
   (5) Muscle tension
   (6) *Sleep disturbance (difficulty falling or staying asleep, or restless or unsatisfying sleep) Note: Sleep disturbance is a symptom of G.A.D.*

D. The focus of the anxiety and worry is not confined to features of an Axis I disorder, e.g., the anxiety or worry is not about having a Panic Attack (as in Panic Disorder), being embarrassed in public (as in Social Phobia), being contaminated (as in Obsessive-Compulsive Disorder), being away from home or close relatives (as in Separation Anxiety Disorder), gaining weight (as in Anorexia Nervosa), having multiple physical complains (as in Somatization Disorder), or having a serious illness (as in Hypochondriasis), and the anxiety and worry do not occur exclusively during Posttraumatic Stress Disorder.

E. The anxiety, worry, or physical symptoms cause clinically significant distress or impairment in social, occupational, or other important areas of functioning.

F. The disturbance is not due to the direct physiological effects of a substance (e.g., a drug of abuse, a medication) or a general medical condition (e.g., hyperthyroidism) and does not occur exclusively during a Mood Disorder, a Psychotic Disorder, or a Pervasive Developmental Disorder. (Generalized Anxiety Disorder)

Note: The sixth criteria for GAD is sleep disturbance. One way some patients react to stress is an increase in their RAS, which presumably contributes to the cause of GAD.

The overactivation of the RAS makes it difficult to deactivate the cortex at desired sleep time. Also, the overactivation of the RAS may interact with sleep. During REM sleep, the cortex is activated and the overactivated RAS may overlay with certain phases of sleep causing the patient to awake during sleep.

The overactivation of the RAS may interact with other vulnerabilities such as Periodic Limb Movements of Sleep (PLMS). A patient may have minimal PLMS in low stress situations. With high stress situations and activation of the RAS, PLMS may increase to a level that interrupts sleep. PLMS are involuntary movements during sleep involving the arms and legs. The patient may have a sense of being restless during sleep or their bed partner might complain of the movements disturbing their sleep.

Meditation and biofeedback may be useful when applied to an overactivated RAS. Other treatments include sedating agents or antianxiety agents that counter the overactivation by the RAS. Also, antidepressants and anticonvulsants have been useful in the treatment of GAD. In this patient, Trazadone, a sedating antidepressant, was useful in treating his insomnia. He also participated in meditation and relaxation therapy with help.

Clinical Example: Psycho-Physiological Problems that Prevent Cortical Deactivation

A 55-year-old working woman who lived alone in an upper middle class neighborhood reported inability to get to sleep. Recently, a neighbor bought a German Shepherd puppy. Late at night, around 10 P.M., the puppy would howl continuously. The patient would lie in bed for one to two hours in total frustration unable to sleep because of the barking. After three weeks, the neighborhood demanded the dog be secured in the owner's house to prevent the neighborhood disturbance. After the barking noise had been eliminated, the patient still could not go to sleep at the desired clock time. The patient developed a psycho-physiological problem that resulted in the inability to deactivate her cortex. This problem could have been avoided if the patient got out of bed when she could not get to sleep. If it takes more than fifteen to twenty minutes to get to sleep, it pays to get out of bed and wait until you feel you can get to sleep.

The "psycho" part of psycho-physiological refers to the negative attitude and "physiological" refers to sleep. Or, negative attitude about going to sleep.

The treatment of the disorder is the same as the treatment to prevent the disorder. If the patient's negative attitude prevents her from deactivating her cortex, then she should get out of bed until she feels tired. The patient should repeat this process until she goes to sleep.

The patient may use medicine to get to sleep. The sedation of the medication offsets the negative attitude about going to sleep. There is risk to this treatment in that the patient may substitute the use of medicine for the negative attitude about sleep. In which case, the patient may develop a dependence on the medicine to get to sleep. This dependence is not addiction, but can be a powerful behavioral force.

There are situations in which noise elimination is not possible. Sometimes, it requires moving to a quiet neighborhood. Some patients find earplugs useful. Or a white noise generator can be a help. A white noise generator is a device that produces all frequencies of sound. When a random noise occurs, it gets lost or drowned out by the white noise. There are natural sounds, like the waves in the ocean breaking on the shore, that approximate white noise.

Clinical Example 3: Drugs that cause problems with cortical deactivation

A 35-year-old woman, executive for a large corporation, married, with one 10-year-old child, complains of insomnia. The patient had increased pressures to perform at work and increased her coffee consumption. With the subsequent development of insomnia, the patient had greater need to increase her coffee consumption in the afternoon and evening. She started to need naps in the afternoon. Since the half-life of coffee is three to seven hours, and the stimulating effects of coffee can last eight to fourteen hours,[2] the patient was instructed to discontinue the use of coffee. It is important to note that some foods, such as grapefruit juice may prolong the effects of caffeine. It just so happens that the patient was on a Weight Watcher's® diet that included grapefruit juice, which probably resulted in an enhanced caffeine effect. Grapefruit inhibits a liver enzyme that metabolizes caffeine and hence increases caffeine concentrations in the blood.

After the patient stopped drinking coffee, there was an adjustment period during which meditation successfully countered her negative attitudes for sleep.

Clinical Example 4: Primary Insomnia

A 25-year-old single female who presented with "I'm a chronic insomniac." Patient stated that she has always had a problem with sleep. She had trouble getting and staying asleep. She had practiced excellent sleep hygiene with little success. She is awakened easily from sleep. If she took medicine with short-lived sedation, she could get to sleep, but would have frequent awakenings. The patient understood that her disorder involved a weak sleep center pull to get her to sleep and to keep her asleep. She was subject to awakening with the slightest movement, sound or light. Her bedroom was like a cave; no light, no sound, temperature was cool with constant temperature and humidity. Her mattress was firm, but not too hard to avoid tactile stimulus movement. She avoided stress and had a job that was easy for her. She avoided interpersonal relationships as even positive emotions could stimulate her cortex and keep her awake all night. She was chronically sleep deprived and depressed. She was lonely because of social isolation. In fact, two years ago, she attempted suicide by overdose.

Chronic insomnia has profound effect on the personality of the patient. Insomnia itself causes depression. The chronic frustration causes demoralization. It is clear that as one approaches the treatment of chronic insomnia or primary insomnia, psychological help is necessary to unlearn maladaptive habits of life.

The first consideration in primary insomnia is to practice good sleep hygiene. In this case, the patient is well informed and practices excellent sleep hygiene. When she has an emotional problem, she does not stay in bed and ruminate about it. She gets up and does some activity until she feels tired. She avoids naps, because the build up of a sleep debt tends to increase the pull to sleep.

The treatment of primary insomnia is not easy. Each person responds to different medications differently. And, more than one medication is usually necessary. The basic medication objectives are to promote getting to sleep, staying asleep and have restorative sleep without side effects of medication. To achieve normalization of sleep in primary insomnia is not easy!

In this case, the patient did fairly well on Klonopin for sedation and Mirapex to suppress restlessness. Psychological therapy helped to reverse her social isolation and to facilitate interpersonal communication. Note: Lunesta, Ambien and Sonata has been shown to be effective for primary insomnia.

Clinical Example 5: Chronic Insomnia

A 50-year-old white, obese male presented with chronic insomnia. The patient tended to fast during the day to lose weight and overeat at night. When the patient would recline, he would notice mild chest pain. The pain would be so severe he could not initiate sleep. The patient's internist, after performing a gastroscopy, diagnosed esophagitis secondary to an incompetent esophageal-gastric value. The patient after reclining would have gastric acid irritate his esophagus causing pain.

The internist sent the patient to a nutritionist and Weight Watchers®. The patient had no snacks after dinner that might stimulate gastric acid. The patient was given a gastric inhibitor pill at bedtime to limit gastric acid secretion. The head of the patient's bed was elevated to promote gravity drainage of gastric acid through the stomach. The patient was given a gastric motility stimulator to promote the emptying of his stomach. After the patient's medical condition was stabilized, his sleep improved.

The patient developed psycho-physiological insomnia secondary to his inability to sleep. Medication and good sleep hygiene helped this problem.

---

[1] American Psychiatric Association: *Diagnostic and Statistical Manual of Mental Disorders*, Fourth Edition, Text Revision. Washington, DC, American Psychiatric Association, 2000.

[2] *Sleep Medicine*, Kryger, Roth & Dement, pg. 1188.

Chapter 5

Melatonin Secretion (Step 2)

"One hour's sleep before midnight, is worth two after."

PROVERB

"Turn the hey deftly in the oiled words and seal the hushed casket of my soul."

JOHN KEATS
TO SLEEP

"Melatonin is the key that opens and shuts the sleep center's door."

ROBERT A. WILLIAMS, M.D.

The brain is an "isolated" system. There is no direct connection to the outside world. The brain creates a "virtual" representation of the outside world. Reality, as we experience it, is a fabrication of the brain. Sleep provides the gas to run the "reality" machine, the brain.

Melatonin is one of three physical steps that are needed to get to sleep. The sleep center provides the pull to the sleep center control area. Melatonin is thought to be the "key" that opens the sleep center door. Also, melatonin needs to be present during sleep or the sleep center door may slam shut and the patient will wake up, unable to return to sleep. As described in Chapter 3, the three elements required to get to sleep are: (1) deactivate the cortex, (2) release melatonin and (3) the pull to sleep caused by low neurotransmitter reserve.

Melatonin is one of the key elements in the brain that allows for the entrainment of sleep. Entrainment means the timing of sleep occurs cyclically during the night. For simplicity, I am referring to melatonin only as the key element which opens the sleep center door. In fact, there are a multitude of complex generators which relate to the entrainment of sleep.

Melatonin is a hormone that is made from a neurotransmitter, serotonin. Serotonin is made from the amino acid L-tryptophan. Amino acids are the building blocks of protein. An example of a source of protein is meat. When proteins are digested in our gastrointestinal tract, amino acids are released into our bloodstream. The basic building blocks of protein are amino acids.[1] Sources of L-tryptophan include turkey and milk. The old wives tale of using warm milk at bedtime for insomnia has a rational basis in fact. Warming milk helps breakdown the proteins in milk releasing L-tryptophan. L-tryptophan has a calming effect (assists in deactivating the cortex) and can be converted to melatonin.

Figure 5-1: Creation of Melatonin

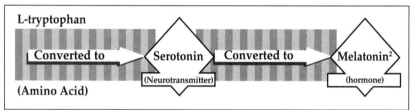

Hormones and neurotransmitters are substances that allow nerve cells to communicate with other cells. Neurotransmitters involve short distances between cells and immediate effects. Hormones are discharged in the blood and involve longer distances between cells and relatively slower effects.

The following are clinical examples of disorders of melatonin secretion (and associated generators of behavior related to sleep onsite disorder).

1. Delayed sleep phase syndrome.
2. Advanced sleep phase syndrome.
3. Jet lag.
4. Aging.
5. Shift work.

Basically the three mechanisms to get to sleep are a checklist to make sure conditions are right to transfer control from the frontal executive area (awake behavior) to the sleep center. The executive function asks the question "Is it safe to go to sleep?" Melatonin release asks "Is it nighttime?" The sleep center asks "Is there a need for sleep?"

Note, the second step in getting to sleep relates to the timing of sleep, i.e., sleep occurs at night (entrainment).

Physiological Checklist for Getting to Sleep

1. Is it safe to go to sleep?
   ☐ Yes – deactivate cortex
   ☐ No – maintain cortical activation

2. Is it dark or nighttime?
   ☐ Yes – release melatonin
   ☐ No – Delay release of melatonin

3. Is there a need for sleep (i.e., is the neurotransmitter gas tank low)?
   ☐ Yes – pull to sleep—turn off histamine release.
   ☐ No – await need to sleep

We normally think of light entering our eyes as exclusively creating vision. In fact, light affects other bodily functions such as pupil size and sleep.

Figure 5-2: The Eye

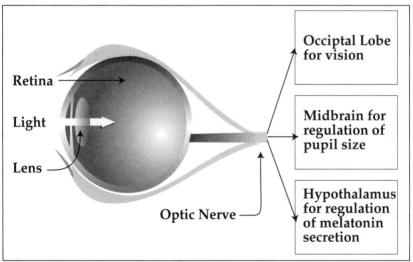

The retina translates light into nerve signals that the brain integrates into meaningful information. Since the brain has no direct connection to the "outside world," it reconstructs information to create an "awareness." Brain reality is the "real" virtual reality.

The retina converts light into nervous system signals.

Melatonin is a substance that is synthesized and released from the pineal gland. Since melatonin signals cells at a distance, it is a hormone.

The diencephalon is a mass of gray matter (brain cells) in front of the midbrain. The top part of the diencephalon contains a diverticulum (out pocketing) called the pineal gland. The cells in the pineal gland (pinealo-cytes) contain and release melatonin.

There is a connection between the hypothalamus (suprachiasmatic nucleus) and the epithalamus (pineal gland). The suprachiasmatic nucleus connects with the retina of the eye. Thus, one can see the anatomical connections between the eye, which senses light, and the discharge of melatonin from the pineal gland.

The release of melatonin is stimulated by darkness and/or by melatonin itself. Light suppresses melatonin secretion.

Hormones are substances that allow brain cells to communicate with each other at a distance. Melatonin is a substance that permits sleep during the night (i.e., opens the sleep center door). Melatonin may also be involved with other functions in the brain. When communication is close-up involving a synaptic cleft (space between cells), the substances are called neurotransmitters. Note: melatonin is also a neurotransmitter in the brain. As a neurotransmitter, melatonin has functions other than sleep.

During the day, the melatonin tank is filled up. When the melatonin level reaches a certain threshold, darkness stimulates the release of melatonin. Thus, two conditions are needed for melatonin release: (1) melatonin tank level and (2) darkness. When the melatonin tank gets too full it overflows, then one can sleep even with lights on. Once melatonin is released, melatonin itself will stimulate melatonin release. Thus, in extreme situations, mechanisms can be overridden, such as the inhibition of melatonin by light.

There are two aspects for the release of melatonin.
   (1) Sensitivity to darkness for the release of melatonin.
   (2) Threshold needed in the melatonin tank for release of melatonin.

The sensitivity to the release of melatonin varies with each individual. Some individuals known as night owls have a delayed release of melatonin. Night owls are able to stay up late because the release of melatonin (and other associated mechanisms) is delayed. The patient is unable to adjust to normal sleep time because the release of melatonin is unable to adjust to normal sleep times.

Figure 5-3: Mechanism of Melatonin Release

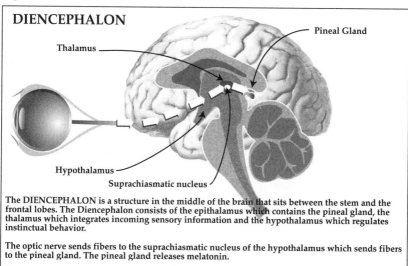

The DIENCEPHALON is a structure in the middle of the brain that sits between the stem and the frontal lobes. The Diencephalon consists of the epithalamus which contains the pineal gland, the thalamus which integrates incoming sensory information and the hypothalamus which regulates instinctual behavior.

The optic nerve sends fibers to the suprachiasmatic nucleus of the hypothalamus which sends fibers to the pineal gland. The pineal gland releases melatonin.

The Diencephalon is a structure in the middle of the brain that sites between the brain stem and the frontal lobes. The top part of the Diencephalon is the epithalamus which contains the pineal gland.

The optic nerve sends fibers to the suprachiasmtic nucleus of the hypothalamus which sends fibers to the pineal gland. The release of melatonin is inhibited by light.

When the release of melatonin is delayed, a person can't get to sleep until late night or early morning. If a person gets up to go to work within a few hours after sleep initiation, he will be sleep deprived. If the process continues, the sleep deprivation will be additive leading to severe impairment. This disorder is called the delayed sleep phase syndrome (DSPS), meaning sleep is delayed from desired clock time.

If, on the other hand, a person who has DSPS is allowed to sleep late in the morning, he will not be sleep deprived. It is the timing of sleep in delayed sleep phase syndrome that causes problems, not the sleep itself.

The timing of sleep is also disrupted in advanced sleep phase syndrome (ASPS). In ASPS, melatonin is discharged earlier than the desired clock time. There is a high sensitivity to darkness or the melatonin tank fills up to a threshold level earlier than desired clock time. The individual can get to sleep easily, but runs out of melatonin early in the morning. These people have early morning awakening and can't get back to sleep. If the person goes to bed early, he/she will get a normal amount of sleep. Usually the person fights going to sleep until the desired clock time and thus with early morning awakening, becomes sleep deprived.

It may be that the trigger for the release of melatonin is defective with either DSPS or ASPS. Normally, when the melatonin tank reaches a certain level, darkness will trigger melatonin release. The trigger for melatonin release may be too early in ASPS. The trigger for melatonin release may be too late in DSPS.

As teenagers, DSPS individuals easily stay up late during slumber parties. Usually the DSPS teenager is the last to go to sleep and the last to wake up. In the case where a teenager can't stay awake during a slumber party, he may reflect an ASPS. Melatonin is secreted early in the evening and the teenager experiences irresistible sleep, while the other teenagers can manage to stay up late watching videos.

The melatonin "tank" may vary in size. A small melatonin tank may fill up to threshold levels early and lead to early melatonin release (ASPS). (Threshold levels means the melatonin tank is filled up enough that darkness stimulates the release of melatonin.) A large melatonin tank may take longer to fill up to threshold levels and lead to delayed melatonin release (DSPS).

Or, the competency of the tank may be a factor (i.e., when the tank is partially full, it may develop leaks). The release of melatonin will stimulate the further release of melatonin. This phenomena occurs with aging. As a person ages, melatonin leaks out earlier, thus people go to bed earlier as they age. Middle-aged people go to bed on time. Old people go to bed early. Young people tend to go to bed late.

Seasons can affect sleep because the length of daylight changes with seasons. In the summer, the length of day is longer and in the winter, the length of day is shorter. In the case of delayed sleep phase syndrome (DSPS), where there is a delay in the release of melatonin, winter time (shorter days) helps to encourage earlier release of melatonin. Since darkness encourages the release of melatonin, winter time tends to help the DSPS individual. On the other hand, the DSPS person is made worse with summer because the longer days tend to suppress melatonin secretion.

The opposite is true with ASPS patients. The patients are worse in the winter because the release of melatonin is early or advanced. The early darkness of winter reinforces the already early release of melatonin. Summer time helps the ASPS patient, because the longer days tend to suppress melatonin secretion to a later time.

As a review, in delayed sleep phase syndrome the melatonin secretion is delayed and in advanced sleep phase syndrome melatonin secretion is too early in the evening. The result of abnormal melatonin secretion is abnormal timing of sleep in relationship to desired sleep time.

There are many changes in sleep as a result of the aging process.[2] The enzymes that fill up the melatonin tank are reduced so that there is less melatonin available for sleep. Melatonin tends to leak out of the melatonin tank at an earlier time at night. The elderly tend to go to bed earlier and have less efficient sleep (sleep efficiency is the percent of time sleeping after getting to sleep). The elderly tend to run out of neurotransmitter gas during the day and needs naps to function. Of course, if the elderly sleep too much during the day there will be no drive to sleep at night. There is a need to balance nap times during the day and ability to function, with the need to be tired at night and the need to consolidate sleep.

Because young persons have large reserves of melatonin, there is more flexibility of sleep patterns. For instance, if a young person misses three hours of sleep during the week, they can sleep in on Saturday or Sunday. A middle-aged person can't "sleep in," usually because the middle-aged person runs out of melatonin and wakes up (i.e., the middle age person does not have the reserve as a young person).

Elderly persons have even fewer melatonin reserves. In order for the elderly to be maximally functional, they can't miss sleep nor naps. In fact, acute confusional states, delirium or sundown syndrome are caused in part by sleep disturbances. Also, note that in elderly patients, long-acting melatonin is recommended. One dose of slow-release melatonin by mouth at bedtime is all that is required. Melatonin stimulates the release of melatonin. In the case of the elderly, where melatonin reserves are low, a slow-release of melatonin makes sense, so that melatonin is available over the entire night.[3] Remember, melatonin is the key that keeps the sleep center door open for sleep.

Jet lag is a sleep disturbance that interferes with normal daytime functioning secondary to crossing several time zones. The mechanism of jet lag is thought to be secondary to entrained (entrained means sleep is synchronized with day and night) biorhythms that need to readjust to a new pattern of day and night. The suprachiasmatic nucleus is a pacemaker for the sleep/wake cycle. The suprachiasmatic nucleus has an intrinsic sleep/wake cycle that is influenced by light and darkness, such that sleep is entrained or occurs at night.

If a person travels eastward, darkness comes sooner than "home" time. Melatonin secretion is accustomed to a later darkness and a later secretion pattern. The melatonin tank is not full enough for darkness to trigger the release of melatonin. The person is unable to go to sleep at desired clock

time. When the person awakes in the morning, he is sleep deprived because of late sleep onset. This is similar to the delayed sleep phase syndrome (DSPS). The average person can adjust one hour per night or can
advance the melatonin secretion toward desired clock time about one
hour per night. Bright light early in the morning shuts off melatonin secretion and allows the melatonin tank to fill up sooner in the nighttime
so darkness will trigger off melatonin secretion at an earlier time.
Melatonin may be given by mouth at night to stimulate the release of
melatonin. Even though the melatonin tank is not full enough for darkness to stimulate the release of melatonin, melatonin can stimulate the
release of melatonin.

There are three variables involved with melatonin secretion:
1. Light and dark.
2. Mechanism of melatonin release (suprachiasmatic nucleus inherent
    rhythm).
3. Melatonin itself.

In the case of the primary disorders of timing of sleep, DSPS and ASPS,
it is the mechanisms of sleep that are abnormal in relationship to light and
dark. In the case of jet lag, changes in work shifts and seasonal changes, it
is light and dark changes in relationship to normal melatonin secretion.

In the case of DSPS and ASPS, we try to adjust the mechanisms to correspond to light and dark. In the case of jet lag, shift changes and seasonal effects, the mechanisms are normal. It is a matter of the normal systems adjusting or changing to a new light/dark pattern.

In the case where a person is traveling west, darkness comes later compared to home time. Melatonin is accustomed to secretion earlier. The
melatonin tank may fill up and overflow before darkness. Or, sleep onset
may be before desired clock time. The person can get to sleep without
problems. The person may awake early because the melatonin tank runs
low. A person can take melatonin when he awakes so he can continue to
sleep. This is similar to ASPS and corrects itself about one hour per night.
Because people do not have trouble getting to sleep, this disorder is not as
troublesome as when traveling east.

Figure 5-4: Jet Lag Created by Traveling East or West

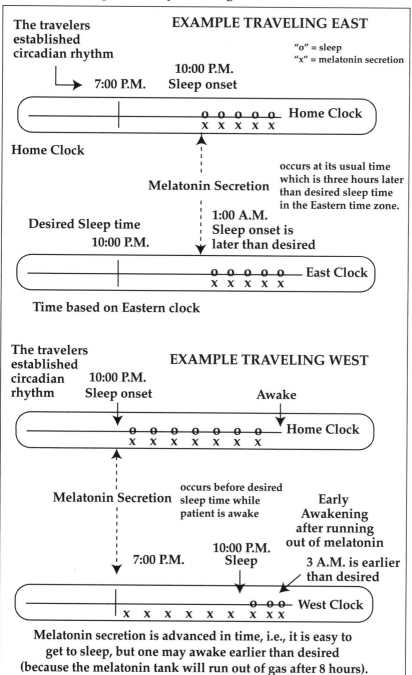

The travelers established circadian rhythm

EXAMPLE TRAVELING EAST

"o" = sleep
"x" = melatonin secretion

7:00 P.M.

10:00 P.M.
Sleep onset

o o o o o   Home Clock
x x x x x

Home Clock

Melatonin Secretion

occurs at its usual time which is three hours later than desired sleep time in the Eastern time zone.

Desired Sleep time
10:00 P.M.

1:00 A.M.
Sleep onset is later than desired

o o o o o   East Clock
x x x x x

Time based on Eastern clock

The travelers established circadian rhythm

10:00 P.M.
Sleep onset

EXAMPLE TRAVELING WEST

Awake

o o o o o o o   Home Clock
x x x x x x x

Melatonin Secretion

occurs before desired sleep time while patient is awake

Early Awakening after running out of melatonin

7:00 P.M.

10:00 P.M.
Sleep

3 A.M. is earlier than desired

o o o   West Clock
x x x x x x x x x

Melatonin secretion is advanced in time, i.e., it is easy to get to sleep, but one may awake earlier than desired (because the melatonin tank will run out of gas after 8 hours).

Travelers are frequently sleep deprived. The pull to pay back their sleep debt may override the tendency to have early morning awakening. Typically a traveler will say, "When I travel west, my sleep is normal" and "When I travel east, then I experience jet lag."

Principles related to melatonin tank:
1. The melatonin tank fills up during the day. It takes approximately sixteen hours to reach a threshold where darkness can stimulate the release of melatonin.
2. If darkness does not stimulate the release of melatonin, the melatonin tank will overflow and the release of melatonin will stimulate the release of melatonin.
3. As the melatonin levels lower during the night, a threshold is reached where light can inhibit the release of melatonin and thereby cause a person to wake up.

Summary
1. *Melatonin* is a hormone that promotes sleep during darkness (entrains or synchronizes sleep to occur at night).
2. *Melatonin* is the second step in a three-step process that is needed for a person to get to sleep. Melatonin is the key that opens the sleep center door.
3. If *melatonin* secretion is delayed at night, sleep is delayed. If sleep is delayed enough to disturb daytime functioning, then it is called **Delayed Sleep Phase Syndrome (DSPS).** Otherwise, we call the person a night owl (a variation of normal).
4. If *melatonin* secretion is advanced to an earlier time at night, then the urge to sleep is advanced compared to desired sleep time. When melatonin secretion begins early, then the melatonin tank runs out of gas early and causes early morning awakening. If this melatonin secretion pattern causes daytime disturbances in functioning, then it is called **Advanced Sleep Phase Syndrome (ASPS).**
5. The release of melatonin is not just related to abnormal release mechanisms seen in DSPS and ASPS. Abrupt changes in day and night in relationship to the usual times of melatonin secretion can cause insomnia as seen in jet lag, seasonal changes and shift work. A change in the timing of release of melatonin takes about one hour per day.
    A person traveling east will have a sleep time that is later than desired sleep time. Sleep time is synchronized with his/her home clock.

Thus, it will be difficult to go to sleep. Melatonin, as a supplement, can be taken orally at bedtime to stimulate the release of melatonin in order to hasten sleep onset.

A person traveling west will feel tired before desired clock time. Sleep onset usually will occur without problems. Early morning awakening may occur because the melatonin tank runs out of gas early. Melatonin may be taken if early morning awakening occurs to facilitate sleep until the desired awake time later in the morning.

6. Shift work has the same effect as travel (i.e., adjustment of suprachiasmatic nucleus to new light/dark pattern).
7. There are three normal ways melatonin is released:
   - Darkness stimulates melatonin release (if the melatonin tank is full enough).
   - Melatonin stimulates the release of melatonin.
   - The overflow of the melatonin tank causes the release of melatonin independent of light/dark patterns.
8. With aging, the production of melatonin decreases and the release of melatonin is earlier in the evening. Aging causes earlier sleep and decreased sleep efficiency. Melatonin supplements may help to increase sleep efficiency and provide more restorative sleep in the elderly.
9. The suprachiasmatic nucleus has an intrinsic rhythm that regulates the sleep/wake cycle. This cycle is modified to correspond to light and dark (i.e., entrained by the secretion of melatonin).

Figure 5-5: Sleep/Wake Cycle Mechanisms and Abnormalities

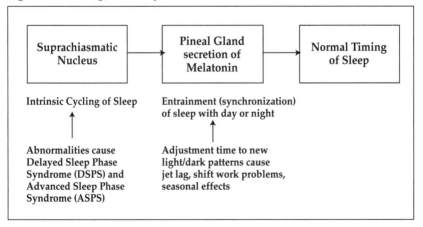

Clinical Sample 1: Delayed Sleep Phase Syndrome

The patient is a 16-year-old male who was sent to the high school counselor because of lack of motivation and poor grades. The teachers noted the patient tended to nod off during class. The patient was thought to be uninterested in school and lacking motivation. His teachers were insulted by his sleeping in class, thinking that he was not interested in their lectures. The patient was referred for attention deficit disorder because of his inability to sustain attention.

When interviewed, the patient did not satisfy the DSM IV criteria for Attention Deficit Disorder (ADD). It became evident when queried about sleep, the patient had a sleep disorder. The patient had a seven-year history of inability to go to sleep at desired clock time. The usual sleep time was 2 or 3 A.M. In spite of good sleep hygiene, including cool room, meditation tapes, quiet and dark room, and taking over-the-counter medication, the patient could not get to sleep before midnight. The patient's school times required him to arise at 6:30 A.M. leaving him sleep deprived. As the week progressed, the patient became more and more sleep deprived. Many times, he could not go to school on Fridays. The patient's weekends were full of sleep time as the patient tried to pay back his sleep debt. The patient's father had similar sleep problems that interfered with his high school career. His father did better academically in college where he could arrange his schedule to have afternoon classes only, thereby sleeping late in the morning allowing for normal sleep time. His father got better with age. Sleep normally advances with age making DSPS better.

The patient satisfied the criteria for Delayed Sleep Phase Syndrome (DSPS):
1. Chronic inability to initiate sleep at desired clock time.
2. Chronic failure of medication to induce sleep.
3. When allowed to sleep, sleep was normal.
4. No obvious psychiatric disorders that might interrupt sleep onset such as mania or anxiety, or substance abuse such as cocaine.

The patient was treated with supplemental melatonin at night to facilitate the release of melatonin. Remember that melatonin is the key that opens up the door of the sleep center. A "brite light" was used in the morning to suppress melatonin secretion. Use of the brite light in the morning suppresses melatonin secretion and tends to preserve the remaining melatonin in the melatonin tank. Presumably, by stopping melatonin secretion, the patient's melatonin tank would fill up to threshold levels earlier in the evening allowing for earlier sleep time.

With a chronic insomnia problem, the patient developed a very negative attitude about sleep. A sedating agent and meditation were used to counter the patient's psycho-physiological disorder. With effort and good sleep hygiene, the patient was able to get to sleep before midnight.

His teachers and counselors were educated about his Delayed Sleep Phase Syndrome. His grades improved dramatically as his sleep improved. Remember, the purpose of sleep is to make neurotransmitter gas to run your brain engine the next day.

Other methods to treat DSPS include chronobiology. The patient darkens his room so **no** light enters. The patient stays awake until 6 A.M. then sleeps. The next day 9 A.M. and each successive day, sleep time is advanced 3 hours. Chronobiology works, but small disruptions in sleep may require a need to repeat the entire process. The process may be impractical for many patients.[4]

Clinical Example 2: Advanced Sleep Phase Syndrome

The patient is a 42-year-old female who complained of early morning awakening. The patient complained of progressive early morning awakening over the past three years. Her past history included inability to stay awake late as a teenager. The patient reported being tired and sleepy early in the evening (6 to 7 P.M.). The patient would fight going to sleep in order to be with her husband until 11 P.M. Frequently, the patient would go to the movies and discover she slept through the entire movie.

The patient satisfied the criteria for Advanced Sleep Phase Syndrome (ASPS):
1. Chronic history of difficulty staying awake.
2. No substance use that account for early evening sedation.
3. If patient goes to bed early, sleep is normal (i.e. restorative).
4. With age, there is a tendency to go to bed earlier (i.e., melatonin leaks out of the melatonin tank earlier). With aging there is a normal advancing of sleep onset, thus making ASPS worse.

Note, the pattern of ASPS is that as a teenager, the patient went to sleep on time (i.e. unable to voluntarily stay awake). As the patient aged, sleep time advanced earlier and earlier. Also, awake time advanced to an earlier time. As a result of this process, the patient had early morning awakening. If a patient resists going to sleep early in the evening, he/she will become sleep deprived.

The treatment of ASPS includes using a bright light in the evening to suppress melatonin secretion until later at night. By suppressing melatonin secretion, the melatonin tank stays fuller before the patient goes to sleep. Thereby, with more melatonin available, the patient is able to sleep longer.

Another treatment of ASPS is to use supplemental melatonin when the patient awakes early in the morning. The melatonin would promote sleep and promote the release of melatonin. The melatonin tank would start to fill up later in the morning, and thus, the melatonin tank would not fill up to threshold levels until later in the evening.

The use of "Brite Light" and melatonin corrected the patient's problem.

Additional history included no history of a psychiatric disorder that may have caused early morning awakening such as major depression.

Clinical Example 3: Jet Lag

A 50-year-old female flew to Germany for a three-week tour of Europe (the trip of a lifetime). The patient found she could not go to sleep until 2 A.M., which was her home normal sleep time. The patient had read *Brain Basics: Sleep* and was prepared. She brought melatonin and a sedative agent to treat her jet lag. The sedative agent was to deactivate her cortex, which was activated by the excitement of her trip and strange and noisy environment. The melatonin was used to induce earlier release of melatonin. Four days into her trip, the patient's sleep normalized.

Clinical Example 4: Aging

The patient was a 75-year-old male who complained of being tired all day in spite of taking naps during the day. The patient had a five-year history of progressive worsening of intermittent sleep.

There are several changes in sleep that occur with aging:
1. Sleep time is earlier because the melatonin tank leaks out melatonin earlier in the evening.
2. The size of the melatonin tank is smaller, so that total sleep time is reduced.
3. The secretion of melatonin may be episodic resulting in intermittent awakening during sleep.
4. The number of restorative enzymes is reduced thereby decreasing sleep efficiency (i.e., it takes longer to fill up the neurotransmitter gas tank).

The approach to the sleep disturbances of the elderly is multifaceted, as one can imagine there are many ways that sleep can go wrong.

Sleep hygiene is important in that one wants to support normal sleep mechanisms as much as possible. Sleep hygiene includes regular bedtime, cool room, avoid large meals at bedtime, quiet environment, comfortable bed and avoid stimulant drugs.

Naps during the day are okay if they are not excessive. In other words, if naps deliver the gas (neurotransmitter) to the engine (nerve terminal), they will a have a revitalizing effect (power nap). If on the other hand the naps are long, the deep sleep will start to fill up the neurotransmitter gas tank, and the elderly patient will have no pull to get to sleep in the evening.

For the elderly who have prominent melatonin secretion problems, supplemental slow-release melatonin is recommended. The melatonin stimulates the release of melatonin and the slow-release continues this process through the night providing more efficient sleep.

As patients age, muscle tone decreases, fat/muscle ratio increases, among other things. As a result, it is important to query for sleep apnea, restless leg syndrome and REM sleep disorder.

Most elderly patients take five to ten drugs per day. Examination of drugs that might affect sleep adversely is important.

As organ systems fail, the brain fails. The purpose of all organ systems is to support the brain. An example is a 75-year-old male who smoked for 40 years and has chronic obstructive pulmonary disease (i.e., it is hard for the patient to get oxygen into his body). The low oxygen will affect his brain diffusely, which is called encephalopathy. Sleep centers are commonly affected by encephalopathy causing intermittent sleep and reversal of circadian rhythm. The treatment includes aggressive treatment of the medical disorder causing the encephalopathy and in this case, oxygen supplement facilitated sleep.

In summary, evaluating and treating sleep disorders of the elderly is complex. It involves:
1. Understanding the changes of sleep physiology with aging.
2. Evaluation of patient for primary sleep disorders.
3. Evaluation of patient for medical disorders that can cause encephalopathy.
4. Use of sleep hygiene and appropriate medication.
5. Evaluation of effects of other medication on sleep.

Clinical Example 5: Shift Work
The patient is a 35-year-old male who works for a company that has round-the-clock production of ammonia nitrate. The union contracted with the company that all laborers would be treated equally and fairly. All laborers therefore worked two weeks on one shift, then advanced to another shift in a

continuous manner. When the patient finished his graveyard shift at 7 A.M., he was unable to go to sleep. He became sleep deprived and eventually developed a depressive illness.

The first focus was providing the patient with a proper sleep environment. His bedroom was darkened so that not one ray of light entered. The temperature was regulated to keep the room cool. And, noise was kept at a minimum. The patient was given supplemental melatonin when he returned home at 8 A.M. to facilitate melatonin release. Eventually, the patient was able to adjust to his rotating shifts.

Note that companies are discovering that is better to have set regular shifts. Rotating shifts creates a great amount of physiological stress in workers who are constantly adjusting to a new shift.[5]

It is important to note that on an individual basis, people have varying capacities to acutely alter their sleep/wake cycles. Age decreases circadian flexibility.

---

[1] Melatonin, Circadian Rhythms and Sleep, *New England Journal of Medicine 2000;* 343:1114–1116.

[2] Insomnia and Sleep Complaints: What is Normal in the Older Adult? Melinda S. Lantz MD, *Clinical Geriatrics,* Vol 10, Number 5, May, 2002.

[3] Haimov I, Lavi P, Landon M, ef Malatonin replacement therapy of the elderly insomniacs. Sleep. 1995; 18:598–603.

[4] Arch. General Psychiatry 1981; 38:737–746.

[5] *Shift Work, Circadian Disruption and Consequences* by Naomi L. Rogers Ph.D. and David F. Dinges, Ph.D., TEN, 2001; 3(9):54–94.

Chapter 6

The Pull to Sleep (Step 3)

"Sleep, dear Sleep, sweet harlot of the senses, Delilah of the spirit."
CHRISTOPHER MARLEY 1890–1957

"Sleep creates the neurotransmitter gas that runs the brain engine."
ROBERT A. WILLIAMS, M.D.

The pull to sleep is the sleep center's way of communicating to the frontal lobes the need to sleep. When neurotransmitters and energy levels are low (i.e., neurotransmitter gas levels are low), the urge to sleep occurs. This is the third step in the three steps needed to get to sleep.
1. Deactivate the cortex.
2. Release of melatonin.
3. Low neurotransmitter levels that result in the pull to sleep.

Frontal lobe executive function is the main controller of the brain during the awake state. The sleep center in the hypothalamus and associated structures is the main controller of the brain during sleep states. The sleep center shifts the metabolic gears of the brain cells from awake state metabolism to restorative state metabolism. Restorative state metabolism involves paying back energy debts and production and delivery of neurotransmitters to the nerve terminals for awake state behavior.

The sleep center has two main functions:
1. Gain control from the frontal lobes.
2. Initiate and maintain a metabolic algorithm that ultimately restores metabolic and neurotransmitter reserves to the brain (i.e., stages of sleep).

The sleep generator of behavior is in the hypothalamus and associated structures in the brain. The purpose of the sleep generator of behavior is to maintain metabolic and neurotransmitter homeostatis for normal brain function during the awake state. Survival and reproduction are the primary functions of the brain. Sleep leaves the human being vulnerable. Thus, sleep is necessary in spite of its dangers to survivability.

The sleep center communicates the need to sleep by creating a pull to sleep or urge to sleep. The frontal lobes reflect the pull to sleep in the awareness center (i.e., instinctive awareness). The frontal lobes may resist the urge to sleep or comply. For instance, a person driving may be tired and have the urge to sleep. The frontal lobes will try to reject the urge to sleep as unsafe. Unfortunately, many persons succumb to the urge to sleep while driving, which is a major cause of accidents on our highways.

The brain is a giant energy-consuming machine. The brain can't simultaneously produce energy and utilize energy.

The sleep generator turns off awake functions:
1. Decreasing frontal lobe control
2. Decreasing temperature
3. Decreasing cortical activation (decreasing RAS and decreasing histamine release)
4. Decreasing spinal reflexes
5. Decreasing movement

During sleep, the sleep generator turns off the gas to the brain engine and body engine in order to produce gas during sleep to run the brain and body engines the next day.

After the sleep generator turns off awake functions, the sleep generator turns on sleep functions. The sleep functions relate to restoring the brain with energy and neurotransmitters for awake functioning.

The pull to go to sleep is related to two functions carried out by the sleep center. The first is to deactivate the cortex by turning off the RAS (Reticular Activating System) and other activating systems. The second is to pull control from executive functions to the sleep center control. Normally, when we are awake, executive function of the frontal lobes is in control. When we sleep, the sleep center is in control. Awake behavior is primary behavior because awake behavior relates to survival and reproduction. Sleep behavior is secondary behavior, but essential for life sustenance. Without neurotransmitters and energy, the brain engine can't operate normally or at all during the awake state.

The frontal lobes during the awake state are activated by two mechanisms:
1. Brain stem activation via the reticular activation system (RAS). The neurotransmitters include norepinephrine and dopamine.
2. Sleep center activation via orexin/hypocrin hormonal systems. The neurotransmitter is histamine.

The sleep center transmits the urge to sleep by turning off the histamine activation to the frontal lobes and decreasing RAS activation. Note that antihistamines such as Benadryl® are used to induce sleep. Benadryl® blocks the activating effects of histamine at the histamine receptor (antihistamine) causing sleepiness.

It is interesting to note that there other neurotransmitters that activate the cortex of the brain such as acetylcholine (Acetycholine is a neurotransmitter with multiple functions depending on the location in the brain. Acetylcholine tends to have an activating effect on the cortex of the brain). Acetylcholine activates the entire cortex, but more specifically the hippocampus related to memory function. The two main neurotransmitters relating to the pull to sleep are histamine and norepinephrine/dopamine. During deep sleep seratonin levels rise and during REM sleep, acetylcholine levels increase.

Four clinical examples of pull-to-sleep disorders are:

Too much pull to sleep:
1. Sedation from drugs or alcohol
2. Primary hypersomnia

Too little pull to sleep:
3. Excessive daytime napping decreases nighttime pull to sleep
4. Primary insomnia is too little inherent capacity to pull to sleep relative to cortical activation

Clinical Example 1: Too Much Pull to Sleep

24-year-old white male, unmarried with a history of chronic alcoholism. Patient was a "functional alcoholic" who worked at a factory from 7 A.M. to 4 P.M. After work, on a daily basis, the patient would go to a local bar and drink until late evening. The patient's chronic alcoholism tended to disrupt his sleep. The patient would take naps at work whenever possible. One night while driving home, he had an irresistible urge to sleep. The patient lost control of his car, hit a tree and was killed instantly on impact. Drugs that sedate, such as alcohol, tend to magnify the pull to sleep. The combination of the normal pull to sleep late at night and the sedation of the alcohol can cause too much pull to sleep and is a leading cause of death on the highway.

Clinical Example 2: Too Much Pull to Sleep

40-year-old chronically-tired patient who felt the urge to sleep all of the time. The patient never felt rested. The patient's sleep was unremarkable in that no abnormalities were noted except that total sleep time was increased, and the patient did not feel rested after a full night's sleep. The patient was diagnosed with primary hypersomnia meaning his restorative enzyme capacity was low. He was unable to fill his neurotransmitter gas tank because of a low capacity to produce neurotransmitter gas and energy. The patient was placed on Modafinal to try to block the pull to sleep with some help. Primary insomnia is a difficult problem to treat.

Clinical Example 3: Too Little Pull to Sleep

The patient is a 30-year-old female with three children; ages 5, 7 and 9. The patient complained of insomnia, specifically the inability to get and stay asleep at night. For several years while raising her children, the patient would take naps during the day to make up for caring for her children at night. The patient got into the habit of napping during the day. One can see how multiple napping during the day might fulfill her sleep needs (i.e., by nighttime her neurotransmitter and energy reserves would be high). Thus, the sleep center had very little pull to sleep. The patient followed a sleep guide with gradually reducing her daytime napping to zero. Her nighttime sleep began to consolidate and eventually returned to normal. It is obvious that not all mothers who nap end up with insomnia after their children begin normal sleep/wake cycles. Basically, some persons have vulnerabilities in the sleep/wake cycles that are not obvious until a stressor brings the vulnerability out.

Other Clinical Examples

There are other disorders that affect too little pull to sleep such as aging and too much pull to sleep such as narcolepsy. They are discussed in other sections.

S E C T I O N   3

RESTORATIVE SLEEP

Chapter 7

The Sleep Center (Introduction to the three steps needed to get restorative sleep)

"Sleep and watchfulness, both of them when immoderate constitute disease."
HIPPOCRATES (C.460BC–C.377BC) GREEK PHYSICIAN
APHORISMS, II

"An imbalance between sleep and awake states causes the brain to fail."
ROBERT A. WILLIAMS, M.D.

The sleep center is a diffuse area of the hypothalamus and brain stem that controls sleep. The sleep center coordinates:

1. When we begin and end sleep.
2. How long we sleep.
3. The measurement of neurotransmitter levels and energy levels and assigns subjective awareness that reflects adequacy of sleep and/or the need for sleep.
4. The on/off mechanism that controls other generators of behavior such as:
   - Spinal reflexes
   - Body temperature
   - Cortisol secretion
   - Frontal lobe activation/deactivation
   - Others

It is presumed that the main goal of sleep is to restore energy and neurotramsitter reserves in the brain. The strategy of the brain is to shut down energy utilization, so that energy can be shunted to the brain for restorative purposes.

1. The cortex energy utilization slows down during sleep.
2. Body metabolism slows down during sleep.

5. There are some classifications of sleep that divide sleep into non-REM sleep and REM sleep. Non-REM sleep is a light sleep and slow wave sleep, both of which are characterized by slow waves. Light sleep has 20 to 50 percent of the EEG record being high voltage slow waves with K-complexes and/or spindles (bursts of fast waves). Deep sleep is defined as more than 50% of the EEG record consists of high voltage slow waves. REM sleep is characterized by an activated EEG record. REM sleep produces low voltage fast waves and other associated features such as rapid eye movement. During REM sleep, the eyes may move together from side to side in a rapid fashion. The eye is a dipole that means the eye has separation of positive and negative electrical charges. The front of the eye (cornea) is positively charged compared to the back of the eye (retina) that is negatively charged. During REM sleep, movement of the eye creates an electrical field that is recorded from electrodes placed on the temples of the patient.

6. The sleep center coordinates the restorative process. The first half of sleep is dominated by deep sleep that creates the neurotransmitter gas. The second half of sleep is dominated by REM sleep that delivers and packages the neurotransmitters at the nerve terminal. The final step in the restorative process readies the brain for human behavior the next day.

7. The sleep center utilizes two mechanisms to gain control of frontal lobe activity.
    a. Turns the RAS down which results in decreased dopamine and norepinephrine activation of the frontal lobes.
    b. Turns histamine activation of the frontal lobes off.

Note there are three systems that activate the cortex depending on function.

1. Dopamine and norepinephrine (both from the brain stem) activate the frontal lobes for the purpose of environmental interaction and planning and execution of tasks.
2. Acetylcholine neurotransmitters (from basal forebrain) activate the frontal lobes and other areas of the cortex for memory function.
3. Histamine neurotransmitters (from the hypothalamus) activate the frontal lobes related to sleep control.

Brain wave patterns reflect sleep states and awake states. The awake state involves low voltage fast brain waves that indicate independent activity in the cortex. The frontal lobes are the most active part of the brain because the frontal lobes orchestrate the *activity of other* cortical regions in an attempt to be adaptable to content-of-life activities.

The last recent phase of animal evolution created the human brain. The human brain is an add-on phenomena. Genetically, the human brain is 95 percent similar to the ape brain. The last 5 percent that was added to the ape brain is the Doral Lateral Prefontal Cortex (DLPC). When one views the human brain from the side, it is quite evident that the frontal lobes are large. The dorsal area of the frontal lobes (e.g. the top part) reveal an enlarged area, DLPC, which is easy to see. It is not hard to imagine where evolution added the last phase of human brain development. The DLPC contains awareness and executive function that posses added cognitive ability and ability to plan and execute complex tasks. Sleep is an instinct and human sleep patterns are similar to other primates.

Although we do not actively think during sleep, the brain actively processes information during sleep. Part of sleep processing of information is creating structural memory (permanent) from biochemical memory made during the day. Memory processing during sleep creates associations between memories and may be the basis of creating insight for problem solving.

When the sleep center takes control from the frontal lobes, the low voltage fast activity of the cortex stops and is replaced by high voltage slow waves. Hence, we have what is called slow wave sleep. It is thought that during the awake state the independent activity of the cortical neurons tend to cancel each other out and produce low voltage fast activity as seen on the EEG. During sleep, the awake activity of the cortical neuron is turned off. Control is taken from the frontal lobe executive function to the sleep center. The sleep center switches the cortical neuronal metabolism from use (awake) to restorative (sleep). Since the cortical neurons are under the control of the sleep center, they don't operate independently. As a result, the cortical neurons operate in synchrony under the control of the sleep center and produce high voltage slow waves.

I propose for heuristic purposes, that light sleep is for transporting amino acids to the neurotransmitter factory—the brain wave pattern consists of high voltage slow waves (>20 percent–<50 percent of the recording are slow waves) and waves unique to light sleep, K-complexes and spindles (unique brain wave patterns). Deep sleep, the making of neurotransmitters, consists of high voltage slow waves (>50 percent of the recording are slow waves).

REM sleep is for transporting and activating the neurotransmitters at the nerve terminal. During REM sleep, as neurotransmitters are readied at the nerve terminal, there is slight overflow of neurotransmitters into the synaptic cleft (the space between brain cells). Suddenly, the cortex produces low voltage fast activity similar to the awake pattern. Vivid dream states occur during REM sleep as a result of this phenomena. One could conceptualize loss of slow wave activity during REM sleep because of the cortical activation from the overflow of neurotransmitters being readied at the nerve terminal.

There are two basic ways that sleep center operations can be disrupted.

1. *Fragment sleep*—In other words, activate the cortex and pull control away from the sleep center, so that the sleep center can't do its job.
2. *Block the sleep centers capacity* to provide restorative sleep within the sleep center. There are two basic pathological processes that can block restorative processes:
    *   Block the progression from light sleep to deep sleep as seen with sleep apnea or restless leg syndrome or from deep sleep to REM sleep as seen in narcolepsy.
    *   Slowing of enzyme activity so that the production of neuro-transmitters and energy is slowed as seen with primary hypersomnia, major depression and chronic fatigue syndrome.

In the case in which a patient has chronic depression that is treatment-resistant, a sleep disorder should be considered. Studies of treatment-resistant depression have shown that up to 40 percent of treatment-resistant patients have a sleep disorder that when diagnosed and treated will have a greater response to their antidepressant medications.

The sleep center is programmed (algorithm) to guide the progression of sleep through the different stages.

REM is rapid eye movement sleep. Non-REM sleep is light sleep and deep sleep.

Figure 7-1: Table of Percentage Stages

	Stages	Approximate Averages
	Wakefulness <5%	Percent of Total Sleep Time
non-REM Sleep (75–80%)	Stage 1 – 2–5% Stage 2 – 45–50%	> 50% *Light sleep* (amino acid transport stage)
	Stage 3 – 3–8% Stage 4 – 10–15%	> 25% *Deep sleep* (making neurotransmitter)
REM	REM – 20–25%	> 25% *REM sleep* (deliver neurotransmitter to nerve terminal)

I use the following metaphor to illustrate the restorative process that occurs during sleep. Light sleep is the crude oil stage or the transport of amino acids to the factory of the brain cell (ribosomes). This is much like pumping crude oil from the ground and transporting the crude oil to the gasoline factory (cracking plant). Deep sleep is the production of gasoline from the crude oil. In the brain cell factory, neurotransmitters are made from amino acids (components from our diet). REM sleep is the transport of the gasoline to the filling station and the delivery of the gas to the engine. In the brain cell, the neurotransmitter is transported to the nerve terminal (filling station) and readied for use by the formation of neurotransmitter vesicles. Neurotransmitter vesicles are packages of neurotransmitters that are readied for release to produce human behavior. The final stage of readying the neurotransmitter for use is like the fuel pump pumping gasoline to the engine of a car.

Figure 7-2: 3 Steps for Restorative Sleep

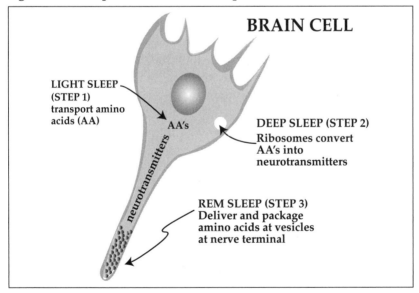

Note: The first half of sleep is mainly slow-wave sleep. The second half of sleep is REM-dominated. The brain cells make the neurotransmitter gas in the first half of sleep, then deliver the neurotransmitter gas to the nerve terminal during the second half of sleep.

The polysomnolgram (PSG) does not define a sleep disorder. PSG does help to define sleep states such as light sleep, deep sleep and REM sleep. The PSG is part of a large database that includes the following data to evaluate a sleep problem:

1. Subjective reports of patient:
    - Onset of sleep problem
    - Family history
    - Sleep diary of patterns of sleep
    - Drug use
    - Medical and psychiatric history
    - Longitudinal history of sleep—example: has sleep problem progressively worsened?
2. Polysomnography: Poly means many measurements; somnography means taken during sleep. Polysomnography measures brain waves, muscle activity, air flow through the mouth and nose, diaphragmic movement, oxygen levels, EKG (electrocardiogram) and eye movement.
3. Physical examination.

Summary of Sleep Center:
1. The brain has two control centers. Awake control center is in the frontal lobes to allow for adaptable behavior in terms of survival and reproduction.
2. The sleep center to provide for the restorative needs of the brain (i.e. the production and delivery of neurotransmitters to the nerve terminals and energy for awake behavior). Sleep is involved with converting biochemical memory to structural memory.
    The sleep center:
    - Turns off awake behavior and turns on sleep behavior.
    - Coordinates through different steps (i.e., stages of sleep) the production and delivery of neurotransmitters to the brain terminal.
3. The brain engine runs on neurotransmitter gas made during sleep.
4. There are three steps to restorative sleep:
    - Light Sleep—transporting of amino acids
    - Deep Sleep—production of neurotransmitters
    - REM Sleep—deliver neurotransmitters to nerve terminal
5. In general, we make neurotransmitter gas during the first half of sleep (deep sleep) and we deliver the gas to the nerve terminal during the second half of sleep (REM sleep). When we sleep, we cycle through the three stages of sleep in a regulated fashion. The first half of sleep is dominated by slow wave sleep. The second half of sleep is dominated by REM sleep. In other words, the percent of REM sleep compared to slow wave sleep increases through the night. Frequently, this is the reason we awake dreaming.

Each of the following three chapters will examine disorders that involve each of the three stages of restorative sleep.

Chapter 8

Light Sleep (Step 1)

"Sleep's the only medicine that gives ease."

SOPHOCLES (C.496BC–406BC) GREEK DRAMATIST PHILOCTETES 766.

*"In order to cope with stress, our executive function needs
neurotransmitter gas produced during sleep."*

ROBERT A. WILLIAMS, M.D.

L ight sleep, is the first step in the restorative sleep process which includes:

1. Light sleep
2. Deep sleep
3. REM sleep

Restorative sleep begins after the brain has finished the checklist of three elements in order to get to sleep:
1. Deactivate the cortex. (Is it safe to sleep?)
2. Melatonin secretion. (Is it dark or nighttime?)
3. Pull to sleep. (Is there a need for sleep?)

Light sleep begins when the normal awake record electroencephalogram (EEG) is replaced by slow waves. When a person is resting and not actively thinking about anything, alpha waves occur in the back of the head. This is a relaxed state of the awake brain. Executive function of the frontal lobes is in control. As the person goes into light sleep, alpha waves breakup and go away. As the sleep center gains control, the alpha waves are replaced by slow waves. Unique to light sleep are spindles and K-complexes. Spindles are short bursts of fast waves and K-complexes are a combination of a slow wave followed by a burst of fast waves. Light

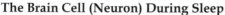

sleep consists of approximately 50 percent of the sleep record. The record during light sleep is less than 20 percent slow waves.

The Brain Cell (Neuron) During Sleep

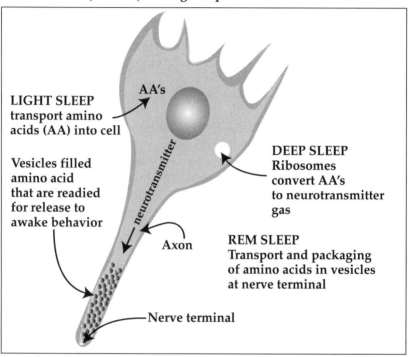

Note that there are three steps in the restorative process. The first step, light sleep, is to transport the amino acids for use in the ribosomes, the neurotransmitter factory. I liken this process to the delivering of crude oil to a gasoline plant. Crude oil represents the amino acids and gas, the neurotransmitters.

Approximately 50 percent of sleep is light sleep. During light sleep, the individual is the least vulnerable to environment threats of the three stages of sleep because muscle tone is maintained and the person is easily aroused.

Figure 8-1: Sleep Disruption Options

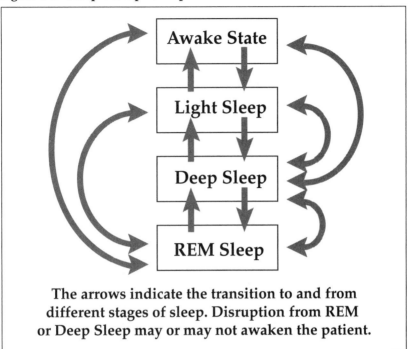

The arrows indicate the transition to and from
different stages of sleep. Disruption from REM
or Deep Sleep may or may not awaken the patient.

After a disruption from light sleep, awakeness occurs. As you can see from the above figure that awakeness is the only arousal option from light sleep. Whereas deep sleep or REM sleep can be interrupted without awakening the patient.

Five situations that may disrupt light sleep:
1. Environmental noise is more likely to alert a person in light sleep compared to other steps of sleep.
2. Stress is likely to intercede during light sleep and awaken a patient.
3. Snoring or movement from a bed partner is likely to awaken a patient from light sleep.
4. Movement of arms or legs as seen in Restless Leg Syndrome more easily awakens a person from light sleep.
5. Physical ailments that create discomfort or pain may awaken a person from light sleep.

Clinical Example 1: Light Sleep

34-year-old female complained of interrupted sleep with tiredness and the need to nap all day. Since being married, her husband gained more than forty pounds and recently began snoring loudly. The patient was instructed to sleep in another room until her husband's snoring was corrected. The patient's sleep resumed to a normal sleep pattern. One's bed partner's sleep problems may affect the other partner's sleep, as in this case. The husband had a sleep study showing significant sleep apnea. The husband went on a diet and used the CPAP (Continuous Positive Airway Pressure) machine. After the patient's husband's problem was corrected (i.e., elimination of noise), then the patient's sleep normalized. *Light sleep is affected by environmental stimuli such as sound.*

Clinical Example 2: Light Sleep

54-year-old male complained of interrupted sleep with the need for daytime napping. The patient had a history of gastritis with esophageal reflux. The patient had a bad habit of eating a large meal before bedtime. The pain of his esophageal reflux would cause the patient to awaken during light sleep. The obvious treatment for this disorder was to avoid large meals or snacks at bedtime and to use antacids or medicines that decrease acid secretion. After the patient modified his eating habits, his sleep normalized. *Light sleep is affected by internal stimuli such as pain.*

Clinical Example 3: Light Sleep

10-old male who was sent to his school counselor because of inability to stay awake in class. The child lived in a very poor area of town and his parents were drug addicts who were in and out of jail. The child's living environment was horrible including very unsanitary conditions. It was noted that he had insect bites on his legs and arms. The child said his mattress was infected with fleas. The outhouse was infested with mosquitoes. The child had interrupted sleep because of his insect bites and itching. There were many other factors that affected the child's sleep including party noise, gunshots, fear and starvation. A city social worker found a friendly and supportive foster home for the child and his sleep improved. Counseling helped the child adjust. *Because light sleep is affected by environmental stimuli, sleep problems can be the presenting complaint of severe social problems.*

Clinical Example 4: Light Sleep

40-year-old divorced female with three children complained of intermittent awakenings with worry. The patient had no trouble getting to sleep.

The patient had work and financial stress. She was tired all day. The patient satisfied the DSM IV criteria for General Anxiety Disorder (GAD). Note that GAD may interfere with getting to sleep, but it can also interrupt sleep. The anxiety related to stress can awaken a person in Step 1 light sleep. The patient was sent to counseling for stress management which helped her sleep. *Light sleep can be interrupted by psychological stress.* Yoga and relaxation techniques can also be useful.

Clinical Example 5: Light Sleep

50-year-old female just reached menopause and complained of intermittent awakening at night. Her husband of twenty-five years stated she had some restlessness, but after menopause her legs moved with "vigor." And, in fact, he had trouble sleeping because he was being kicked so much. Periodic limb movement of sleep (PLMS) may worsen after menopause as many disorders do. The patient was referred to her gynecologist for possible estrogen replacement therapy (ERT). After being treated with a dopamine agonist, the patient's PLMS resolved. *PLMS can interrupt any step of sleep, but Step 1 sleep is the most sensitive to movement.*

Summary of Light Sleep

Light sleep is just what it says it is, "light sleep." The majority of sleep, approximately 50 percent, is spent in light sleep. The person in light sleep is more responsive to his environment which has an evolutionary protective value. Environmental noise, snoring from a bed partner, stress, restless legs or medical reasons are common problems that interrupt light sleep. *Correcting the problem that interrupts light sleep involves removing the stimulus that creates the interruption such as noises, pain, anxiety or restlessness.*

Note: Light sleep, is the first step in the restorative process of sleep.

Chapter 9

Deep Sleep (Step 2)

"That sweet, deep sleep, so close to tranquil death."

VIRGIL
AENEID, VI

"Frontal lobe awareness is disconnected during sleep, providing calmness."

ROBERT A. WILLIAMS, M.D.

"Laugh and the world laughs with you; snore and you snore alone."

ANTHONY BURGESS (BORN 1917) DUTCH NOVELIST & CRITIC.
INSIDE MR. ENDERBY

"Noise disrupts sleep and is very aversive to persons trying to sleep."

ROBERT A. WILLIAMS, M.D.

To review, the brain is the organ system of behavior.

Behavior is anything that reflects brain activity. There are three behaviors of the brain that reflect the electrochemical properties of the brain:

1. Overt behavior is the outward behavior of the brain we see or perceive without special equipment.
2. Electrical behavior of the brain is measured by the electroencephalogram (EEG). Sleep is the only normal behavior that is measured by the electroencephalogram. Because the brain produces electrical fields, it also produces magnetic fields that can be measured and can interact with the TMS (transcranial magnetic stimulator) in the treatment of depression.

3. Neuroendocrine behavior is measured by hormones which is the brain's connection to the body (i.e., mind-body connection).

As a person transitions from awake to light sleep to deep sleep, the electroencephalogram transitions from low voltage cortical (fast) waves to high voltage slow waves. High voltage slow waves reflect sleep center control over the cortex. The cortex is synchronized to the "beat" of the sleep center creating high voltage slow waves. When the cortex is under control of the frontal lobes, specific areas of the cortex are activated for awakeness, planning and executing tasks. When the frontal lobes are in control the brain wave pattern is low voltage fast activity.

Deep sleep, is slow-wave sleep. There are many things that distinguish deep sleep from light sleep. Characteristics of deep sleep include:

1. Interruption of deep sleep can occur without awakening (i.e., transition from deep sleep to light sleep). Whereas interruption of light sleep will cause awakening.
2. The electroencephalogram shows >20 percent slow waves (i.e., slow wave sleep or predominance of slow waves).
3. Muscle tone decreases (i.e., there is a relative paralysis).

Figure 9-1: EEG—Awake and Deep Sleep

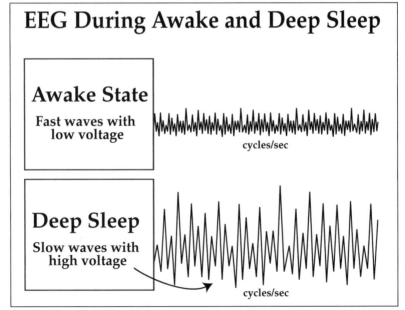

Deep sleep is for the production of neurotransmitters that are needed to run the brain engine (i.e., our personality).

To review, there are three steps in the process of restorative sleep.
1. Light Sleep: transport of amino acids into the cells
2. Deep Sleep: producing neurotransmitters
3. REM Sleep: packaging, delivery and activation of neurotransmitters for awake behavior

There are two main disorders that interrupt deep sleep:
1. Sleep apnea.
2. Periodic Limb Movement of Sleep (PLMS).

   The progression of light sleep into deep sleep is accompanied by a relative paralysis of the muscles of the body. The collapse of the oral airway from the relative paralysis causes a pressure differential between the outer and inner airways. Clinically if the collapse is complete, breathing will cease (i.e. apnea). If it is partial, decreased breathing will occur (i.e. hypopnea). The pressure differential between the inner and outer airway may cause snoring or labored breathing. Depending on the sensitivity of the individual, interruption of deep sleep may occur reverting a patient back to light sleep where muscle tone is restored (e.g. arousal). By restoring muscle tone, the pressure differential will improve and possibly the breathing itself. Note some patients have severe apnea such that the oxygen levels in the blood as measured by pO_2 (partial pressure of oxygen) are low. If PO_2 is low enough for long periods, patients can sustain brain damage from the low PO_2 itself, which is a separate brain insult from sleep deprivation. The heart also may be sensitive to low PO_2 levels leading to cardiac arrhythmias.
   When a patient goes into REM sleep, there is total paralysis and an increase in heart rate that subjects the apneic patient to the greatest cardiac stress. It is not uncommon for the elderly to die during sleep.

Figure 9-2: Brain Cell

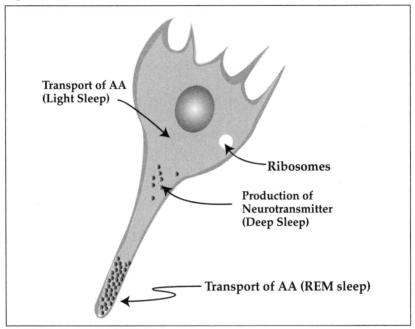

Figure 9-3: Muscle Tone* During Different Stages of Sleep

Sleep Stage	Muscle Tone
1. Light Sleep	High (no paralysis)
2. Deep Sleep	Low (partial paralysis)
3. REM	None (total paralysis)

*Motor (muscle) tone relates to the resting activation of a muscle.

Figure 9-4: Mechanism of Sleep Apnea

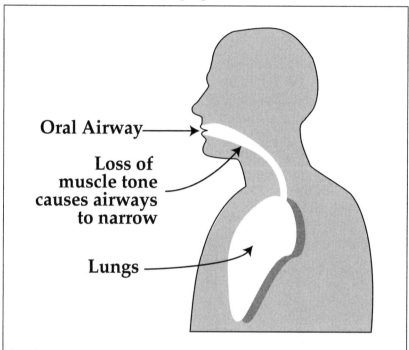

Patients who have sleep apnea are given five therapeutic options that are designed to keep the airway open during deep sleep.

1. Surgery to open up the airway to reduce pressure differentials, such as tonsillectomy.
2. Tracheotomy—surgery to bypass the oral airway all together.
3. CPAP—Continuous Positive Airway Device—a device used to maintain pressure throughout the airway so that there is not a pressure differential during deep sleep (i.e., air splint). By eliminating air turbulance, the arousals that follow the air turbulance are eliminated. Restoration sleep can proceed.
4. Oral airway device that fits into the mouth.
5. Conservative approach consisting of weight loss and positioning during sleep.

Any conditions that affect airway size can contribute to sleep apnea or sleep restrictive disease. The following is a list of some conditions that contribute to airway restriction:

1. Allergies—thickened mucous membranes.
2. Fat—neck fat pushes in on the oral airway.
3. Asthma (narrows airways). Worsens sleep apnea by a separate process.
4. Unusual anatomy of neck such as large tonsils or adenoids or fat deposits.
5. Malpositioning of the tongue that compromises the airway.
6. Chronic obstructive pulmonary disease (COPD) is a decreased ability to move air in and out of the lungs.
7. Other Causes

Figure 9-5: Multimodal Approach to Enhance Airway at Night

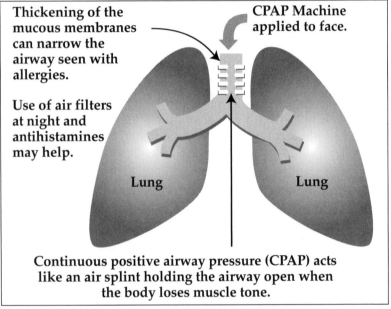

Thickening of the mucous membranes can narrow the airway seen with allergies.

Use of air filters at night and antihistamines may help.

CPAP Machine applied to face.

Lung

Lung

Continuous positive airway pressure (CPAP) acts like an air splint holding the airway open when the body loses muscle tone.

Part of the physical exam for the sleep disorder patient includes the following:
1. Observe for obesity:
   - Fat deposits in the neck can narrow the airway
   - Fat deposits on the chest and abdomen can inhibit breathing capacity (i.e., Pickwickion Syndrome)
2. Observe oral airway:
   - Narrow oral airway
   - Large tongue
   - Large tonsils
   - Enlargement in neck, such as thyroid tumor
3. Observe lung capacity for breathing:
   - Asthma
   - Chronic Obstructive Pulmonary Disease (COPD)
   - Others

Figure 9-6: Recording from Polysonnogram

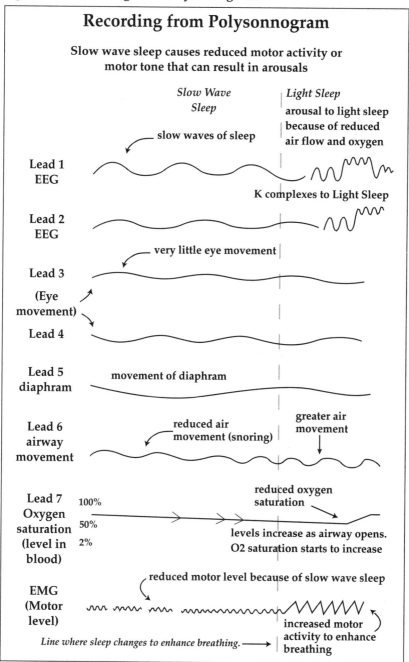

Recording from Polysonnogram

Slow wave sleep causes reduced motor activity or motor tone that can result in arousals

Slow Wave Sleep

Light Sleep
arousal to light sleep because of reduced air flow and oxygen

slow waves of sleep

Lead 1 EEG

K complexes to Light Sleep

Lead 2 EEG

very little eye movement

Lead 3 (Eye movement)

Lead 4

movement of diaphram

Lead 5 diaphram

reduced air movement (snoring)

greater air movement

Lead 6 airway movement

reduced oxygen saturation

Lead 7 Oxygen saturation (level in blood)

100%

50%

2%

levels increase as airway opens. O2 saturation starts to increase

reduced motor level because of slow wave sleep

EMG (Motor level)

increased motor activity to enhance breathing

Line where sleep changes to enhance breathing. ⟶

Principles and Practice of Sleep Medicine, 3rd Ed., Kryga Roth Dement, pg. 844.

Figure 9-6 is a recording from a polysonnogram. The polysonnogram shows the effects of slow wave sleep and light sleep on breathing and oxygen levels in the blood. In the first part of the polysonnogram, the sleep stage is slow wave sleep or deep sleep.

In Deep Sleep, muscle tone is lost, oxygen saturation gradually goes down, breathing volume stops, and snoring begins. As the polysonnogram progresses, the patient reverts to light sleep. EEG shows loss of slow waves (not making neurotransmitters) when sleep changes to light sleep.

In Light Sleep, muscle tone recovers, oxygen saturation increases, breathing volume is restored, and snoring stops. EEG shows arousal to light sleep.

Polysonnography is useful for diagnosing sleep apnea.

By measuring airflow and steps of sleep, one can measure how sleep is interrupted by sleep apnea. Figure 9-6 shows a pattern of oxygen saturation in a patient with severe apnea. The oxygen levels drop from 90 percent to 70 percent. Above 90 percent is normal. Also, one can make a correlation of decreased oxygen saturation and snoring. In light sleep, the increase in muscle tone allows for breathing to resume. Low oxygen levels that occur during sleep apnea can have a direct toxic effect on the brain (hypoxia).

One can see that if deep sleep is interrupted during an (arousal), neurotransmitter gas is not going to be produced. When the neurotransmitter gas level is low, then the patient will feel tired and want to sleep during the day (i.e., daytime hypersomnalance).

Periodic limb movement of sleep (PLMS) can interrupt any of the three steps of sleep. In the case of deep sleep, PLMS may cause deep sleep to revert to light sleep or awaken a patient. PLMS may be part of the restless leg syndrome (see Glossary).

Clinical Example: Deep Sleep

45-year-old white male complained of falling asleep during the day. The patient was an executive of a large corporation and was unable to stay awake during critical meetings. The patient fell asleep while driving and ran into a tree totaling his car. He no longer drives at night for fear he'll fall asleep. He also complained of memory problems and difficulty concentrating.[1]

The above is a typical story for sleep apnea. The patient's polysonnogram showed severe sleep apnea with hypoxic episodes (his blood oxygen levels decreased during his apneic episodes). The patient's hypoxic episodes would explain his decreased capacity to remember things and his decreased concentration.

The patient used a CPAP (continuous positive airway pressure) machine with good results. To reverse the effects of chronic non-restorative sleep, it takes 5 to 10 months or 10 to 20 percent improvement per month[2].

Summary of Deep Sleep

1. Deep sleep produces the neurotransmitter gas to run the brain engine the next day.
2. Muscle paralysis during deep sleep can cause restriction of the airway leading to sleep apnea.
3. Interruption of deep sleep may not awaken the patient. The usual complaint of deep sleep interruption is daytime sleepiness or tiredness, not insomnia.
4. The CPAP machine is used for sleep apnea by providing an air splint to keep the airway open during paralysis caused by deep sleep.
5. PLMS is treated with medicine such as dopamine agonists which inhibit involuntary leg movements during sleep.

---

[1] New England Journal of Medicine, Vol 347, No. 7, Pg. 501.

[2] Dr. Williams' guess.

Chapter 10

REM Sleep (Step 3)

"Sleep is when all unsorted stuff comes flying out as from a dustbin upset in a high wind."

WILLIAM GOLDING (BORN 1911) BRITISH NOVELIST
PINCHER MARTIN

"Awake defense mechanisms may not operate during sleep."

ROBERT A. WILLIAMS, M.D.

"To be, or not to be, that is the question…
To die, —to sleep; —to Sleep!
Perchance to dream: —ay, There's the rub;
For in that sleep of death what dreams may come."

WILLIAM SHAKESPEARE
HAMLET'S SOLILOQUY – ACT III, SC. 1

"REM sleep is necessary for dreaming."

ROBERT A. WILLIAMS, M.D.

The last step of restorative sleep is Rapid Eye Movement Sleep or REM sleep. REM sleep is usually referred to as dream sleep, although vague dreams may occur during other steps of sleep. The purpose of REM sleep is to deliver the neurotransmitter gas to the nerve terminal for use the next day.

Figure 10-1: The Three Steps of Restorative Sleep

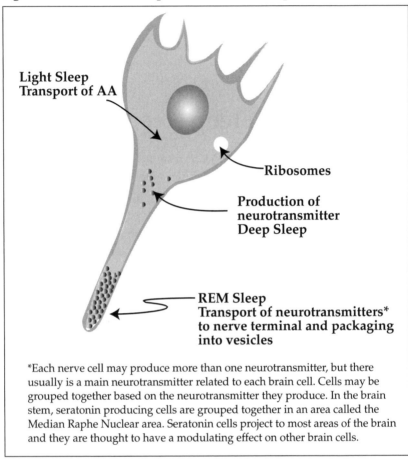

Light Sleep
Transport of AA

Ribosomes

Production of
neurotransmitter
Deep Sleep

REM Sleep
Transport of neurotransmitters*
to nerve terminal and packaging
into vesicles

*Each nerve cell may produce more than one neurotransmitter, but there usually is a main neurotransmitter related to each brain cell. Cells may be grouped together based on the neurotransmitter they produce. In the brain stem, seratonin producing cells are grouped together in an area called the Median Raphe Nuclear area. Seratonin cells project to most areas of the brain and they are thought to have a modulating effect on other brain cells.

When the neurotransmitter gas tank is "full," the hypothalamus will signal "full" to the frontal lobe awareness center. The person will feel rested. The limbic system will reward the person for satisfying the instinct for sleep by a sense of well-being. The person will feel well. On the other hand, when we say "the person got up on the wrong side of the bed," the person did not get adequate sleep and is irritable. Irritability is a form of limbic system punishment, in this case for not having satisfied the instinct for sleep.

The second half of sleep is dominated by REM. Therefore, when patients cut their total sleep time short by watching the late night movie, they are REM sleep deprived. The patient is sleep deprived, but mainly in the REM phase of sleep. Power naps during the day help move the neurotransmitters to the nerve terminal. Self-imposed REM sleep deprivation is the most common disruption of REM sleep.

Narcolepsy is a disease that affects REM sleep. Apparently, the enzymes that move or activate the neurotransmitters are defective. Therefore, there is great pressure to deliver neurotransmitters to the nerve terminal. During the day, the patient may experience sleep attacks, cataplexy (sudden loss of muscle tone), hypnogogic hallucinations and sleep paralysis. These breakthrough symptoms are normal phenomena seen during REM sleep. Scheduled naps during the day help. Medicines that block REM sleep such as Dexedrine® help. Medicines that block the pull to sleep such as Provigil® also may help. Medicines such as sodium oxybuterate push the patient into deep and REM sleep, which helps with daytime sleepiness and decreases catalepsy.

Interestingly, symptoms of sleep disorders can be misinterpreted. Focal cataplexy (loss of muscle tone) can be misinterpreted as a small stroke, or dystonia. REM intrusion during the day (i.e., short intense dreams) can be misinterpreted as hallucinations or attention deficit disorder.

Psychological misinterpretations of sleep disorders also occur. The person with a sleep disorder might be seen as lazy, lacking motivation, disinterested or dumb. If there is not gas to run the brain engine, the brain will not operate normally.

Clinical Example 1: REM Sleep

22-year-old recently married female stayed up late enjoying late night movies and being with her husband. She would awaken tired and needed naps during the day. Her work suffered. She read **Brain Basics: Sleep** and realized that her brain needed neurotransmitter gas. She discussed her needs and her health issues with her husband. They both got to sleep earlier and enjoyed getting REM sleep which predominates in the second half of sleep.

Clinical Example 2: REM Sleep

20-year-old farmer found he drove his tractor into a neighboring farm without remembering what he did. He had a four-year history of falling down with laughter (cataplexy can be triggered by emotion). Cataplexy may precede the onset of sleep attacks in some individuals. The patient awoke at times unable to move his muscles (sleep paralysis). His father was diagnosed with narcolepsy. This is a typical story of narcolepsy which is usually a hereditary sleep disorder. The patient took scheduled naps and used Dexedrine and Provigil to help prevent falling asleep.

Summary of Section 2 and Section 3
Summary of Getting to Sleep and Getting Restorative Sleep

1. There are three steps needed to get to sleep.
   a. deactivation of cortex;
   b. melatonin key and
   c. pull to sleep (low neurotransmitter levels)
2. There are three steps needed for restorative sleep that take place in the sleep center:
   a. Mobilizing amino acids into the nerve cell—Light Sleep
   b. Making neurotransmitters—Deep Sleep
   c. Delivery and activation of amino acids to nerve terminal—REM Sleep
3. Processes that cause disruption from the sleep center to wakefulness usually will result in the complaint of insomnia because the patient associates sleep disruption with being tired the next day.
4. Processes that disrupt the progression of sleep in the sleep center cause daytime hypersomnolance, and frequently the patient is unaware of the cause of his/her sleep problem.
5. The two most common medical problems that disrupt deep sleep are Sleep Apnea and/or Restless Leg Syndrome.
6. The problem that disrupts REM sleep is narcolepsy. Self imposed decreased sleep duration disrupts REM sleep because REM sleep dominates the latter half of sleep.
7. Sleep studies provide data:
   • Time to Sleep—Is there a delay of sleep?
   • Total Sleep Time—Is sleep long enough?
   • Is there interruption of Deep or REM Sleep?
8. Restorative sleep is assessed by three clinical parameters:
   a. When a person awakes do they feel "rested" (the hypothalamus signals "rested" when the neurotransmitter gas tank is full)
   b. When a person awakes, they feel "well" (sense of well-being) the limbic system rewards the person for satisfying the instinct of sleep. When person comments, "They got up on the wrong side of the bed", they are referring to the limbic system punishment (irritability related unsatisfactory sleep)
   c. Restorative sleep allows a person to function during the day with no signs of sleep deprivation such as extreme tiredeness or excessive need for naps.

9. There are 3 steps needed for restoration sleep.
    a. Step 1 is light sleep.
    b. Step 2 is slow wave sleep.
    c. Step 3 is REM sleep.

S E C T I O N   4

Parasomnia, Classification,

and Summary of Sleep

Chapter 11 – Parasomnias

Chapter 12 – Classification of Sleep Disorders

Chapter 13 – Summary of Sleep Principles

Chapter 11
Parasomnias

"It appears that every man's insomnia is different from his neighbors as are their daytime hopes and aspirations."

F. Scott Fitzgerald (1896–1940) US Writer.
The Crack-up, 'Sleeping and Waking'

"Sleep is needed for daytime functioning."

Robert A. Williams, M.D.

Parasomnias is a brief chapter to summarize the concepts and descriptions of the parasomnias. "Para" is a latin derivative meaning alongside or next to. "Somnia" means sleep. Parasomnias are events that occur separately from the normal sleep mechanisms such as sleep walking. The definition of parasomnia is any undesirable motor, verbal or experiential phenomena that occur during sleep. Parasomnic events are *usually* classified as to whether they occur during REM sleep or non-REM (NREM) sleep (NREM sleep is light and slow wave sleep).

Parasomnias are undesirable events that occur during sleep, may also be classified by the type of undesirable event.

Figure 11-1: Types of Parasomnias

MOTOR (movement)	
Normal motor activity seen during the awake state, but abnormal during sleep states	Limb Movement: Walking
Abnormal motor activity seen during the awake state, and obviously abnormal during sleep states	Bruxism (grinding teeth) Dystonia (abnormal posturing) Seizures Combative Behavior
VERBAL (vocal)	
Talking Screaming	
EXPERIENTIAL (what we experience)	
Nightmares Psychosis	

It is thought that the brain states NREM or SWS (deep sleep) and REM sleep relate to the parasomnias that occur during these phases of sleep.

NREM, which includes deep sleep, is a brain state of low capacity for arousal. In the case of NREM sleep arousal parasomnias, the arousal process is not normal or complete. Part of the brain is aroused and part of the brain is not. It is thought that any process that deepens sleep and has the capacity for arousal, can lead to NREM parasomnias. One example is alcohol use. Initially, alcohol is sedating and promotes deep sleep. As alcohol is metabolized out of the body, withdrawal activates the brain and can cause confusional arousals. Another example are deep sleepers, patients who are sleep deprived may experience enhancement of deep sleep. Central nervous system depressants such as barbituates can enhance deep sleep. It is thought that the enhancement of deep sleep may make it difficult to execute the alerting sequence that leads to the awake state, and thereby may cause NREM arousal parasomnias.

Figure 11-2 shows predisposing, facilitating and triggering factors in NREM arousal parasomnia.

Figure 11-2: Triggering Factors in NREM Arousal Parasomnias

Predisposing Factors Genetic factors—family history of same or other NREM arousal parasomnias
Factors That Deepen Sleep (Increase Slow-Wave Sleep or Increase the Difficulty in Awakening, i.e., Arousal) Young age Natural deep sleeper Recovery from prior sleep deprivation Onset of CPAP therapy for obstructive sleep apnea CNS depressant medication (sedatives, hypnotics, alcohol) Fever Hypersomniac period (e.g., in Kleine-Levin syndrome)
Factors That Fragment Sleep Stress Environmental stimuli Endogenous stimuli Pain Pregnancy Stimulants Thyroxine taken in evening Migraine headache Tourette's syndrome
CNS, central nervous system; CPAP, continuous positive airway pressure.[1]

NREM sleep consists of light sleep and deep sleep. Light and deep sleep occur mainly in the first half of sleep for the purpose of producing neurotransmitters. REM sleep dominates in the second half of sleep. Thus, we see NREM arousal parasomnias during the first half of sleep. NREM arousal parasomnias occur mostly during childhood (i.e., the immature brain).

NREM arousal parasomnias consist of the following:

1. Confusional arousals last thirty seconds to five minutes. The person awakes in a *confused* but alert state. Executive function is unable to focus and orient the person. Executive function does not fully develop in the adult brain until age 23. It is not hard to see how executive function in the immature brain might be vulnerable to any alerting or activating process.

2. Sleep terrors last thirty seconds to five minutes. Sleep terrors consist of sitting up during sleep, emitting a cry and showing behavior features of *acute terror*. The person experiencing sleep terrors usually does not remember the terror incident.
3. Sleep walking usually lasts less than fifteen minutes. The person is unaware of his walking, but will awaken in a strange place out of bed or return to bed unaware of the entire incident.
4. Faulty arousal mechanisms may lead to inappropriate confusion, terror or walking during the first half of sleep (NREM sleep).

There are two common REM-related parasomnic disorders:
1. Nightmares
2. REM sleep behavior disorder (RBD)

The following is the Diagnostic Statistical Manual IV Criteria for Nightmare.

DSM IV Diagnostic Criteria for Nightmare Disorder (307.47)

> **A.** Repeated awakenings from the major sleep period or naps with detailed recall of extended and extremely frightening dreams, usually involving threats to survival, security, or self-esteem. The awakenings generally occur during the second half of the sleep period.
>
> **B.** On awakening from the frightening dreams, the individual rapidly becomes oriented and alert (in contrast to the confusion and disorientation seen in Sleep Terror Disorder and some forms of epilepsy).
>
> **C.** The dream experience, or the sleep disturbance resulting from the awakening, causes clinically significant distress or impairment in social, occupational, or other important areas of function.
>
> **D.** The nightmares do not occur exclusively during the course of another mental disorder (e.g., a delirium, Post-traumatic Stress Disorder) and are not due to the direct physiological effects of a substance (e.g., a drug of abuse, a medication) or a general medical condition.
>
> Note that REM sleep increases during the second half of sleep when nightmares occur.

REM sleep Behavior Disorder (RBD) is a condition where REM muscle paralysis is lost and the patient acts out his dreams. The following table lists causes of RBD.

Figure 11-3: Causes of RBD (REM Sleep Behavioral Disorder)

Acute RBD	Etiology
Withdrawal	Alcohol Meprobamate Pentazocine Nitrazepam
Intoxication	Biperiden Tricyclic antidepressants Monoamine oxidase inhibitors Caffeine
Chronic RBD	
Toxic-metabolic	Tricyclic antidepressants Fluoxetine Venlafaxine Selegiline treatment for Parkinson's Disease Anticholinergic treatment for Alzheimer's disease
Vascular	Subarachnoid hemorrhage Vasculitis Ischemic
Tumor	Acoustic neuroma Pontine neoplasm
Infectious, post-infectious	Guillian-Barré syndrome
Degenerative	Amyotrophic lateral sclerosis Anterior/dorsomedial thalamic syndrome (fatal familial insomnia) Dementia (including Alzheimer's disease and diffuse Lewy body disease and corticobasal degeneration) Demyelinating disorder Olivopontocerebellar degeneration Parkinson's disease Progressive supranuclear palsy Shy-Drager syndrome Multiple system atrophy Normal pressure hydrocephalus
Traumatic	Head trauma
Developmental, congenital, familial	Narcolepsy Tourette's syndrome Group A xereoderma pigmentosum Mitochondrial encephalomyopathy
Idiopathic	(See text)[2]
RBD, REM sleep behavior disorder.	

The following table shows the most common features of various parasomnias.

Figure 11-4: Comparison of the Most Common Features of Various Parasomnias[3]

	Confusional Arousals	Sleep Terrors	Sleepwalking	Nightmares	RDB	Complex PS
Time of night	Early	Early	Early to mid	Late	Late	Any
Sleep stage at start	SWS	SWS	SWS	REM	Dissociated REM	Any
EEG discharges	No	No	No	No	No	Usual
Screams	No	Yes	No	Rare	Rare	Rare
CNS activation	Minimal	Extreme	Minimal	Mild	Mild	Mild
Myoclonus	No	No	No	Rare	Common	Rare
Walking	No	No	Yes	No	Rare	Common
Returns to bed	Stays	Stays	Usual	Stays	Unusual	Unusual
Awakens	Uncommon	Uncommon	Uncommon	Common	Common	Common
Duration	0.5–10 min.	1–10 min.	2–30 min.	3–20 min.	1–10 min.	5–15 min.
Confusion (after)	Usual	Usual	Usual	Very Rare	Rare	Usual
Reduced in laboratory	Yes	Yes	Yes	No	No	No
Episodes in wake	No	No	No	No	No	Usual
Age	Child	Child	Child	Adult	Adult	Adult
Genetic transmission	Yes	Yes	Yes	No	No	Rare
Organic CNS lesions	No	No	No	No	Common	Common

CNS, central nervous system; dissociated REM, sleep consisting of REM sleep without atonia; PS, partial epileptic seizures; RBD, REM sleep behavior disorder; SWS, slow-wave sleep (i.e., stages 3 and 4)

Epilepsy: "The sole manifestation of nocturnal seizures may be simple arousal, which may or may not be perceived by the patient. If a sufficient number of arousals occur, the resulting sleep fragmentation will present with symptoms of severe excessive daytime sleepiness. These seizure-induced arousals may be associated with very minor motor phenomena."[3]

Seizures can interfere with sleep during REM or NREM sleep.

To summarize, parasomnias are undesirable events that occur during sleep. The undesirable events can be motor, verbal or experiential.

There are three common NREM parasomnias (usually childhood):
1. Confusional arousals
2. Sleep terrors
3. Sleepwalking

There are two common REM parasomnias:
1. Nightmares
2. REM Sleep Behavior Disorder—RBD (adult)

Other disorders that may be associated with sleep are bruxism (grinding of teeth), enuresis (loss of bladder control), nocturnal paroxysmal dystonia (muscle contractions), primary snoring, migraine headaches and panic attacks.

---

[1] *Principles & Practice of Sleep Medicine,* 3rd Ed. Kryger, Roth, Dement, WB Saunders Co., 2002, pg. 694.

[2] *Principles & Practice of Sleep Medicine,* 3rd Ed. Kryger, Roth, Dement, WB Saunders Co., 2002, pg. 726.

[3] *Principles & Practice of Sleep Medicine,* 3rd Ed. Kryger, Roth, Dement, WB Saunders Co., 2002, pg. 695.

Chapter 12

Classification of Sleep Disorders

"There ain't no way to find out why a snorer can't hear himself snore."

MARK TWAIN (SAMUEL L. CLEMENTS: 1835–1910) U.S. WRITER
TOM SAWYER ABROAD – CHAPTER 10

"For patients that snore, restorative sleep is limited and the pull to sleep is great."

ROBERT A. WILLIAMS, M.D.

Now that you have learned the basic principles of sleep, we are going to study the classification of sleep disorders. We will examine two resources that classify sleep:

1. DSM IV—Diagnostic Statistical Manual IV, which is used by mental health care workers and others.
2. The International Classification of Sleep Disorders that is used by neurologists, sleep specialists and others.

First, we will review the basic principles of sleep:

There are three steps in order to get to sleep
   1. Deactivate cortex
   2. Melatonin key to unlock the sleep center door
   3. Low levels of neurotransmitters that cause the pull to sleep

There are three steps in order to get restorative sleep
   1. Light sleep to transport amino acids into the brain cells
   2. Slow-wave sleep or deep sleep to make neurotransmitters
   3. Rapid eye movement (REM) sleep to move and activate the neurotransmitters for daytime use

All of the classifications of sleep disorders fit into the basic principles of sleep. By applying the basic principles of sleep to the classification of sleep, one can easily understand the classification system.

Diagnostic Statistical Manual IV (DSM IV) Classification of Sleep:
The DSM IV classification lists five disorders of sleep called dyssomnias. The classifications are a list of sleep disorders based on the broad definition of dyssomnia. Dyssomnias are caused by a disturbance in the amount, quality or timing of sleep and are characterized by excessive sleepiness or difficulty in initiating/maintaining sleep (DSM IV p.553)[1]. The following is a list of the DSM IV dyssomnias.

1. *Primary insomnia* is defined a "...difficulty in initiating or maintaining sleep..." (DSM IV p.299) and "not secondary to other mental disorder or any organic factor..." (DSM IV p.301) One might view primary insomnia as a weak sleep generator of behavior.
2. *Primary hypersomnia* involves prolonged sleep episodes with daytime sleepiness or sleep. Apparently, in spite of sleep that appears normal, sleep is not restorative. Other notable behaviors include "sleep drunkenness" and autonomic behavior, such as not being aware of having driven to a particular place.
3. *Narcolepsy* involves the onset of sleep during awake periods. Presumably, sleep suppression mechanisms are defective, which causes the following essential features of narcolepsy:
   - Irresistible attacks of refreshing sleep
   - Cataplexy, or sudden loss of muscle tone
   - REM sleep during transition between sleep and wakefulness, which is manifested by hallucinations or sleep paralysis
4. *Breathing-related sleep disorders* disrupt normal sleep and cause daytime sleepiness. Obstructive sleep apnea, which is accompanied by loss of spinal reflexes, is the most common breathing-related sleep disorder and is caused by paralysis or collapse of the upper airway in susceptible individuals. When the upper airway collapses, air flow may stop or be highly restricted. When oxygen levels drop, the patient is alerted and stops REM sleep. REM sleep deprivation may result in daytime somnolence.
5. *Circadian rhythm disorder* is a recurrent pattern of sleep disruption that results from a mismatch between an individual's endogenous circadian sleep-wake system and exogenous demands regarding the timing and duration of sleep.

The five major dyssomnias from the DSM IV can be viewed from the Williams Brain Model (Figure 12-1).

1. Primary insomnia involves decreased capacity to deactivate the cortex, probably related to a weak sleep center pull to get to sleep. The first step in the process of getting to sleep (e.g., deactivation of the cortex). Relative to the activation of the cortex, the pull to sleep by the sleep center will have varying capacities to getting a person to sleep. Primary insomnia is "primary" in that the primary sleep mechanisms to get to sleep are faulty. Primary Insomnia involves the relative strengths of the activating mechanisms of the cortex (Step 1 in getting to sleep) and the pull to sleep by the sleep center (Step 2 in getting to sleep.)
2. Primary hypersomnia involves too few restorative enzymes. In spite of normal sleep, the person has daytime hypersomnolence, the patient cannot fill up his neurotransmitter tank. Primary hypersonmia involves Step 2 in getting restorative sleep.
3. Narcolepsy involves poor sleep suppression so that during wakefulness the person has sleep attacks, loss of muscle tone (cataplexy) and REM sleep, patient can not deliver neurotransmitter gas to the brain engine. Narcolepsy involves Step 3 in getting restorative sleep.
4. Breathing-related sleep disorders that secondarily prevent restorative sleep. Sleep apnea prevents deep sleep. Breathing related sleep disorders involve Step 2 in getting restorative sleep.
5. Circadian rhythm disorder relates to the melatonin secretion (i.e. the timing of sleep). Circadian sleep disorder involves Step 2 in getting to sleep.

It is easy to see how the five major dyssomnias in the DSM IV fit into the Williams Brain Model of Sleep.

Primary insomnia involves Step 1, ability to deactivate the cortex and Step 3, the pull to go to sleep by the sleep center.

Circadian Rhythm sleep disorders involve the release of melatonin (and associated mechanisms) which is the key that opens the sleep center door (Step 2 in the 3 steps to get to sleep).

In *primary hypersomnia* the reduced numbers of ribosomes make it impossible to make enough neurotransmitter gas. In spite of sleeping a lot, the person always feels tired and somnalant.

Sleep Classification and the Williams Brain Model for Sleep

Figure 12-1: 3 Steps in Getting to Sleep

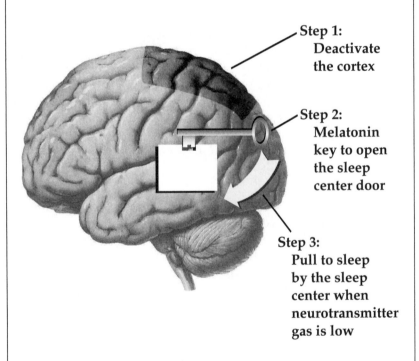

Williams Brain Model

Three Steps To Get To Sleep

Sleep is a process that creates neurotransmitter gas and energy that runs the brain engine the next day.

There are three steps needed to get to sleep.

Step 1:
Deactivate the cortex

Step 2:
Melatonin key to open the sleep center door

Step 3:
Pull to sleep by the sleep center when neurotransmitter gas is low

When a patient is unable to get to sleep he will complain of "insomnia."

Figure 12-2

Williams Brain Model
Three Steps To Get Restorative Sleep

Sleep is the process that creates neurotransmitter gas and energy that runs the brain engine the next day. Restorative sleep occurs when a person awakes feeling rested and feeling well and has a sense of well-being.

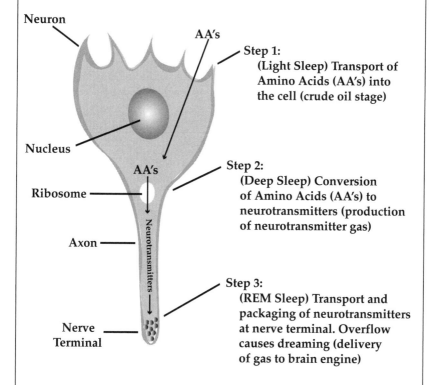

Neuron

AA's

Step 1:
(Light Sleep) Transport of Amino Acids (AA's) into the cell (crude oil stage)

Nucleus

AA's

Step 2:
(Deep Sleep) Conversion of Amino Acids (AA's) to neurotransmitters (production of neurotransmitter gas)

Ribosome

Axon

Neurotransmitters

Step 3:
(REM Sleep) Transport and packaging of neurotransmitters at nerve terminal. Overflow causes dreaming (delivery of gas to brain engine)

Nerve Terminal

When a person does not get Restorative Sleep, they complain of daytime "tiredness" and have propensity to fall asleep (daytime hypersomnolance).

In *narcolepsy* the transport or packaging of neurotransmitters is defective. There is a tremendous pull to get neurotransmitter gas to the brain engine which causes the symptoms of narcolepsy, cataplexy, sleep attacks and hypnogogic hallucinations. In *breathing-related sleep disorders* or *sleep apnea*, the paralysis that occurs during deep sleep causes a narrowing of the airway. The narrow airway causes air turbulence. The air turbulence causes arousals. The person can not get restorative sleep.

The main categories of the classification adapted from the *International Classification of Sleep Disorders*[2] follows:
Dyssomnias
  • Intrinsic sleep disorders
  • Extrinsic sleep disorders
  • Circadian rhythm sleep disorders
Parasomnias
  • Arousal disorders
  • Sleep-wake transition disorders
  • Parasomnias usually associated with REM sleep
  • Other parasomnias
Medicopsychiatric sleep disorders
  • Associated with mental disorders
  • Associated with neurological disorders
  • Associated with other medical disorders

The following are comments concerning the *International Classification of Sleep Disorders* classifications:
• Intrinsic means within the body. Primary intrinsic means a sleep disorder that relates to deficit within the sleep mechanisms. An example is narcolepsy. Secondary intrinsic means a sleep disorder that is secondary to another organ system within the body that interrupts the normal sleep mechanism. An example is sleep apnea.
• Extrinsic means outside of the body. Examples are food allergy insomnia or environment sleep disorder such as loud noises, bright flashing lights or heat. Environmental factors that counter normal sleep mechanisms tend to disrupt sleep.
• Circadian Rhythm sleep disorders are not disorders of sleep itself, but of the timing of sleep and are considered a separate category. Circadian rhythm disorders may be extrinsic such as jet lag or intrinsic such as a genetic predisposition for delayed sleep.

After five years of work, in 1990, the International Classification of Sleep Disorders (ICSD) was published. A revised edition of the ICSD was published in 1997[3].

The International Classification of Sleep Disorders

	Recommended ICD-9-CM No.		Recommended ICD-9-CM No.
Dyssomnias		Sleep-onset association disorder	307.42-5
Intrinsic Sleep Disorders		Food allergy insomnia	780.52-2
Psychological insomnia	307.42-0	Nocturnal eating (drinking) syndrome	780.52-8
Sleep state misperception	307.49-1	Hypnotic-dependent sleep disorder	780.52-0
Idiopathic insomnia	780.52-7	Stimulant-dependent sleep disorder	780.52-1
Narcolepsy	347	Alcohol-dependent sleep disorder	780.52-3
Recurrent hypersomnia	780.54-2	Toxin-induced sleep disorder	780.54-6
Idiopathic hypersomnia	780.54-7	Extrinsic sleep disorder NOS	780.52-9
Post-traumatic hypersomnia	780.54-8	*Circadian Rhythm Sleep Disorders*	
Obstructive sleep apnea syndrome	780.53-0	Time-zone change (jet lag) syndrome	307.45-0
Central sleep apnea syndrome	780.51-0	Shift work sleep disorder	307.45-1
Central alveolar hypoventilation syndrome	780.51-1	Irregular sleep-wake pattern	307.45-3
Periodic limb movement disorder	780.52-4	Delayed sleep phase syndrome	780.55-0
Restless leg syndrome	780.52-5	Advanced sleep phase syndrome	780.55-1
Intrinsic sleep disorder NOS	780.52-9	Non-24-h sleep-wake disorder	780.55-2
Extrinsic Sleep Disorders		Circadian rhythm sleep disorder NOS	780.55-9
Inadequate sleep hygiene	307.41-1	**Parasomnias**	
Environmental sleep disorder	780.52-6		
Altitude insomnia	993.2	*Arousal Disorders*	
Adjustment sleep disorder	307.41-0	Confusional arousals	307.46-2
Insufficient sleep syndrome	307.49-4	Sleepwalking	307.46-0
Limit-setting sleep disorder	307.42-4	Sleep terrors	307.46-1

	Recommended ICD-9-CM No.
Sleep-Wake Transition Disorders	
Rhythmic movement disorder	307.3
Sleep starts	307.47-2
Sleeptalking	307.47-3
Nocturnal leg cramps	729.82
Parasomnias Usually Associated with REM Sleep	
Nightmares	307.47-0
Sleep paralysis	780.56-2
Impaired sleep-related penile erections	780.56-3
Sleep-related painful erections	780.56-4
REM sleep-related sinus arrest	780.56-8
REM sleep behavior disorders	780.59-0
Other Parasomnias	
Sleep bruxism	306.8
Sleep enuresis	780.56-0
Sleep-related abnormal swallowing syndrome	780.56-6
Nocturnal paroxysmal dystonia	780.59-1
Sudden unexplained nocturnal death syndrome	780.59-3
Primary snoring	780.53-1
Infant sleep apnea	770.80
Congenital central hypoventilation syndrome	770.81
Sudden infant death syndrome	798.0
Benign neonatal sleep myoclonus	780.59-5
Other parasomnias NOS	780.59-9

	Recommended ICD-9-CM No.
Sleep Disorders Associated with Medical or Psychiatric Disorders	
Associated with Mental Disorders	
Pyschoses	292-299
Mood Disorders	296-301
Anxiety Disorders	300
Panic Disorder	300
Alcoholism	303
Associated with Neurological Disorders	
Cerebral degenerative disorders	330-337
Dementia	331
Parkinsonism	332-333
Fatal familial insomnia	337.9
Sleep-related epilepsy	345
Electrical status epilepticus of sleep	345.8
Sleep-related headaches	346
Associated with Other Medical Disorders	
Sleeping sickness	086
Nocturnal cardiac ischemia	411-414
Chronic obstructive pulmonary disease	490-494
Sleep-related asthma	493
Sleep-related gastroesophageal reflux	530.1
Peptic ulcer disease	531-534
Fibrositis syndrome	729.1

In summary, the five major dyssomnias as described in the DSM IV can be understood easily in the Williams Brain Model of Sleep.

The ICD-9-CM classification of sleep disorders is also easily understood in the context of the basic principles of sleep.

When approaching any classification of sleep, it is important to know the basic sleep mechanisms:

The Three Steps to Get to Sleep:
1. Deactivate the cortex.
2. Melatonin key to unlock the sleep center door.
3. Pull to sleep.

The Three Steps Needed to Get Restorative Sleep:
1. Light sleep to move in amino acids.
2. Deep sleep to make neurotransmitters.
3. REM sleep to activate and ready neurotransmitters for daytime use.

---

[1] American Psychiatric Association: *Diagnostic and Statistical Manual of Mental Disorders,* Fourth Edition, Text Revision. Washington, DC, American Psychiatric Association, 2000.

[2] *Principles and Practice of Sleep Medicine,* Kryger, Roth and Dement, pg. 547.

[3] *Harrison's Principles of Internal Medicine,* pg. 212.

Chapter 13

Summary of Sleep Principles

"Health is the first muse and sleep is the condition to produce it."

RALPH WALDO EMERSON (1803–1882) U.S. POET AND ESSAYIST.
UNCOLLECTED LECTURES, 'RESOURCES'

"Sleep is necessary for good health."

ROBERT A. WILLIAMS, M.D.

"The overlap of all the generators of behavior in the brain creates our personality or brain engine. Sleep provides the gas to run our brain engine."

ROBERT A. WILLIAMS, M.D.

1. The purpose of sleep is to fill up the neurotransmitter gas tank and energy reserves to run the brain engine during awake hours the next day.
2. Sleep is one of three *Williams' Wells* defining brain stability:
   a. Sleep well
   b. Feel well
   c. Function well
3. Each of the above *Williams' Wells* relates to different ascending levels of brain function. Sleep well relates to the hypothalamus and brain stem, feel well relates to the limbic system and function well relates to the frontal lobes' executive functions.

Figure 13-1: Three Steps To Get to Sleep Sleep

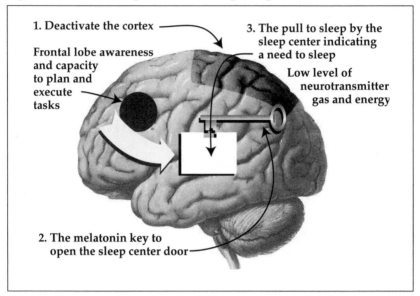

1. Deactivate the cortex

Frontal lobe awareness
and capacity
to plan and
execute
tasks

3. The pull to sleep by the
sleep center indicating
a need to sleep

Low level of
neurotransmitter
gas and energy

2. The melatonin key to
open the sleep center door

Figure 13-2: Three Steps To Get Restorative Sleep

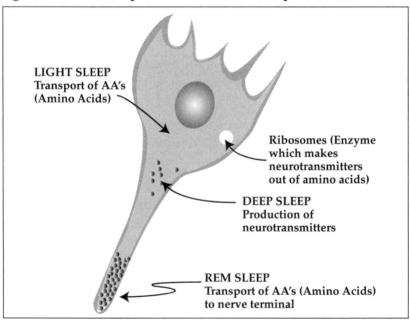

LIGHT SLEEP
Transport of AA's
(Amino Acids)

Ribosomes (Enzyme
which makes
neurotransmitters
out of amino acids)

DEEP SLEEP
Production of
neurotransmitters

REM SLEEP
Transport of AA's (Amino Acids)
to nerve terminal

4. There are three steps needed to get to sleep and stay asleep (See Figure 13-1):
   a. Deactivate the cortex (relax the mind).
   b. Melatonin key to open the sleep center door (release melatonin from pineal gland).
   c. Low neurotransmitter levels (the pull to sleep).
5. Insomnia or the perception one can't sleep properly is caused by the inability to get to sleep or stay asleep. The interruption of one or more of the steps to get to sleep results in the complaint of "insomnia."
6. There are three steps needed to get restorative sleep (See Figure 13-3):
   a. Light sleep—transport amino acids (crude oil stage).
   b. Slow wave sleep—make neurotransmitters (produce the gasoline).
   c. REM (rapid eye movement) sleep—deliver neurotransmitters to nerve terminal (deliver gas to the brain engine).

Table 13-3: Three Steps to get Restorative Sleep

Step 1	Step 2	Step 3
Light Sleep	Deep Sleep (slow wave)	REM Sleep (dream sleep)
Transport amino acids	Produce neurotransmitters	Deliver & package amino acids for use
Pump crude oil	Gasoline production	Deliver gasoline to engine

7. *Daytime sleepiness* is caused by non-restorative sleep. The interruption of one of the three steps in getting restorative sleep may cause daytime sleepiness or tiredness.
8. There are three clinical signs of adequate restorative sleep.
   a. When a person awakes feeling "rested," it is the hypothalamus signaling "full tank of gas" (i.e., no pull to sleep and activation of cortex).
   b. When a person awakes feeling "well," it is the limbic system rewarding the person for satisfying the instinct of sleep.
   c. During the day, the person does not exhibit signs of inadequate sleep such as falling asleep, feeling tired or excessive need for naps.
9. Three common sleep disorders are:
   1) *Primary insomnia* is a weak sleep generator that is affected by other generators of behavior such as obsessive worry. This is an example of inability to deactivate the cortex.

2) *Delayed sleep phase syndrome* is the delayed release of melatonin that prevents sleep at desired clock time. This is an example of inability to open the sleep center door with the melatonin key.

3) *Sleep apnea* is a breathing disorder that prevents restorative sleep. This is an example of blocking neurotransmitter production.

10. Most insomnias that present clinically are primary in that the sleep generator is relatively weak in relation to bad sleep habits or the activation of other generators of behavior (such as anxiety or obsessive worry).

11. Sleep hygiene includes regular sleep hours; quiet, cool room; avoiding stimulants such as caffeine; avoiding alcohol; avoiding sleep associations such as watching television when you go to sleep. Sleep hygiene refers to habits that reinforce the sleep generator's normal sleep mechanisms and are useful to treat primary insomnia.

12. Sleep deprivation contributes to industrial and car accidents, health problems such as obesity and high blood pressure, treatment-resistance to psychiatric problems and to creating psychiatric problems such as depression.

13. Many sleep disorders can be diagnosed by clinical interview, physical examination and a sleep diary. The main diagnostic tool for the diagnosis of sleep disorders is polysomnography, which is a sleep study involving many measurements taken during sleep.

Brain Basics: Sleep—Summary
In general what do we do about sleep disorders (treatment options)?

1. Primary insomnia—Primary goal of therapy is to deactivate the cortex.
   - Sleep hygiene is used to reinforce normal sleep physiology.
   - Sedation with medication is used to deactivate the cortex.
   - Meditation is used to disconnect activating generators of behavior.

2. Psycho-physiological insomnia (negative attitude toward sleep)—Primary goal is to deactivate the cortex.
   - Relaxation tapes are used to decrease anxiety associated with sleep.
   - Meditation is used to undo negative thoughts about sleep.
   - Sedation with medication is to counter anxiety associated with sleep.
   - Sleep hygiene.

3. Delayed sleep phase syndrome—Primary goal is to induce the discharge of melatonin (and associated structures) to open up the sleep center door at an earlier or desired clock time.

- Melatonin by mouth to induce the release of melatonin.
- Light in the morning to stop melatonin discharge so that the melatonin tank fills up sooner at night.
- Chronobiology—reset the melatonin clock by advancing sleep time beginning in the morning.

4. Sleep apnea—Primary goal is to promote normal breathing so that a person acquires restorative sleep (i.e. fills up their neurotransmitter gas tank).
    - CPAP machine—continuous positive airway pressure device to maintain normal breathing that allows for restorative sleep (positive pressure acts as an "air splint"). The air splint holds the airway open during the time of muscle paralysis during deep or REM sleep.
    - Weight loss may help provide a more patent airway during sleep.

5. Fragmented sleep (part of primary insomnia) due to a weak sleep generator pull—Goal is to enhance the sleep generator of behavior pull during sleep to counter fragmentation of sleep.
    - Avoid naps during the day to enhance sleep consolidation at night.
    - Medicines such as Provigil® (Modofinil) blocks sleep center pull to sleep during the day by promoting release of histamine.

6. Restless Leg Syndrome—The purpose of treatment is to suppress leg movement during sleep so that restorative sleep is not interrupted.
    - Dopamine antagonist such as Mirapex® (Pramipexole) and many other medicines have variable effects on suppressing leg movement during sleep. Mirapex suppresses involuntary movements during sleep much like it inhibits tremors of Parkinson's Disease.

7. Insomnia secondary to depression usually causes fragmented sleep and/or early morning awakening. Trouble getting to sleep occasionally occurs.—The primary treatment is to treat the underlying depression after which baseline sleep will resume. Since the response rate to antidepressants is slow, the treatment of insomnia for a depressed patient as a separate issue is usually necessary. In addition, daytime tiredness may need to be treated until the antidepressant works.

The following is a basic algorithm for the treatment of any brain disorder.
1. Survival—try to prevent suicide or accidents.
2. Treat symptoms of illness such as sleep disorder, anxiety, agitation or daytime tiredness.

3. Treat underlying illness.
4. Prevent relapse.

Note: Step 2 recommends the treatment of symptoms of illness such as sleep disturbances. The treatment of insomnia related to depression is to use either antidepressants that provide sedation or add a separate agent that provides sedation at bedtime. The purpose of treatment is to consolidate sleep so that restorative sleep occurs. Escalation of depressive symptoms occurs when the depression causes insomnia. Mania is also accelerated with sleep deprivation. In general, all psychiatric disorders are destabilized by sleep disorders.

8. Fragmented sleep secondary to a medical condition such as asthma— Primary treatment is to treat the underlying medical condition so that baseline sleep occurs. Frequently, medical disorders are treatment-resistant and supplemental sleep aides are necessary.

9. Jet lag is treated depending on the direction one is traveling. Basically, if one has trouble getting to sleep, one takes supplemental melatonin at bedtime. If one has early morning awakening, one takes melatonin upon awakening. Sedative medications can also be used instead of melatonin or in addition to melatonin as the brain adjusts to a new pattern of day and night.

10. Advanced sleep phase syndrome is a condition where melatonin is secreted too early in the evening. The patient runs out of melatonin early in the morning and experiences early morning awakening. Treatment consists of light in the evening to suppress melatonin secretion and the use of melatonin upon awakening.

11. Restorative sleep is assessed by 3 clinical parameters.
    1) When a person awakes they feel rested (the hypothalamus signals "full tank of gas" to run the brain engine).
    2) When a person awakes they feel well. The limbic system rewards the person for satisfying the instinct of sleep.
    3) The person functions normally during the day and there are no signs of sleep deprivation.

Review of Very Common Sleep Problems

1. *Weak sleep generators* that are disrupted by poor sleep hygiene. The solution is to avoid caffeine and alcohol. Avoid exercise at night. Keep a quiet, cool room. Don't go to bed until tired. Use meditation. Possibly use sedating medication.

2. *Stress* induced anxiety, obsessive worry or obsessive thought that activates the cortex. Solution is to work on reducing stress. Use meditation to deal with anxiety and obsessive thoughts. Exercise during the day. Possibly use sedating medication.

3. *Negative attitude about sleep.* If a patient continuously fails to go to sleep, he will develop a negative attitude about going to sleep. The negative attitude in itself can prevent sleep even if the cause of the insomnia is removed. The solution is to not go to bed unless you feel tired or you think you can go to sleep. Do not stay in bed longer than twenty minutes. If you can't get to sleep, then get up and do something then try again when you feel tired. Possibly use sedating medication to counter the activating effects of the negative attitude. Negative attitudes are usually in the form of "I can't go to sleep."

4. *Positive associations* with sleep that disrupt sleep. An example is only going to sleep with the television on. The patient develops such a large association with sleep and the television being on that the patient can't sleep without the television being on. The solution is to avoid going to sleep with associated stimuli.

5. *Delayed sleep phase syndrome (DSPS)* is the inability to sleep at desired clock time due to a delay in the secretion of melatonin. When the patient gets to sleep, he/she will have normal restorative sleep. Sleep needs are not met because the patient will need to get up on time in the morning for school or work. If the patient is allowed to sleep, he/she will sleep until late morning or early afternoon. A mild form of this disorder is commonly termed being a "night owl."

6. *Sleep apnea.* It is important to note that during restorative sleep the body is partially paralyzed and during REM sleep the body is totally paralyzed (atonia). During restorative sleep and REM sleep, one's airway is reduced because the airway partially collapses as a result of the paralysis. If the airway is reduced enough, the air turbulence causes snoring. If the airway totally collapses, then breathing stops (sleep apnea). If the airway is reduced enough or breathing stops, then the brain is alerted and the person awakens or moves to a lighter step of sleep. After the alerting episode, muscle tone increases and allows for enhanced breathing. The person is unable to maintain restorative sleep because every time the patient moves into restorative sleep, breathing difficulties occur and the alerting mechanism causes him/her to move into a lighter sleep.

Clinical Example 1: Delayed Sleep Phase Syndrome:
20-year-old male college student couldn't get up for 8 A.M. classes. He fell asleep during his afternoon classes. He was failing his classes because he couldn't concentrate or stay awake. The patient had similar problems in high school. The patient's mother worked swing shift at the local factory because she needed to sleep in to get enough sleep. The patient tried alcohol and sleeping pills to get to sleep without success. The patient's psychiatric and neurological exams were within normal limits (WNL). All labs are WNL. The patient's sleep normalized with supplemental melatonin at night and bright light in the morning. The patient's performance at school improved greatly.

How can non-restorative sleep interrupt the treatment of depression?

Clinical Example 2:
37-year-old married white female who has 2 children, 5 and 10 years old, complained, "I've been treated with high doses of five antidepressants and none have helped my depression." The patient had no history of drug abuse (a common cause of treatment resistance). Thyroid and sex hormone levels were WNL (another common cause of treatment resistance). Physical exam and MRI of brain were WNL (i.e., she has no neurological abnormalities that might indicate a neurological disorder such as multiple sclerosis).

Psychiatric exam revealed a depressed white female. Body type was obese. Her eyes showed dark circles. She sat with a hunched posture. She appeared tired and sleepy. Affect was constricted. No psychosis was present. She was alert 0x3, but had a difficult time concentrating.

Review of System:
Patient had carbohydrate cravings (carbohydrate cravings are seen with sleep deprivation and depression). Patient felt sleepy all the time and did not feel rested in the morning. Her husband complained of decreased sexual interest (which is seen with depression and non-restorative sleep). Sleep study showed severe sleep apnea, which corrected with CPAP (continuous positive airway pressure) machine. Her depression resolved with continual use of antidepressants and CPAP machine.

The mechanism of treatment resistance is the non-restorative sleep (involves the neurotransmitter gas tank). When a patient does not get restorative sleep, the brain cells are low in all the neurotransmitters. The Prozac or SSRI blocks the re-uptake of serotonin. If the cell is low in serotonin, then the serotonin is not available to be blocked by the anti-depressant.

In summary, sleep is a basic instinct that is needed for normal brain functioning.

Glossary

Advanced Sleep Phase Syndrome (ASPS) — A disorder of the timing of sleep. The patient tends to go to sleep earlier than desired clock time. The patient tends to have early morning awakening as the result running low on melatonin. The patient is sleep deprived or tired as a result of ignoring the pull to sleep during early evening.

Algorithm — A recipe or series/sequence of prescribed events leading to a goal.

Amino acids — Molecules (groups of atoms) that possess a nitrogen atom and acid group. Amino acids are found in many food groups, but are best known as the building blocks of protein. When proteins in our diet are digested, amino acids are released into our blood stream to be used in a variety of ways by our organ systems. One way amino acids are used is to create neurotransmitters by brain cells.

Autonomic Nervous System — Autonomic refers to a division of the peripheral nervous system. The peripheral nervous system is "peripheral" to the central nervous system (CNS) the brain. The autonomic nervous system (ANS) tends to have independent control of its motor functions (smooth muscle of lungs, heart, intestine, salivary glands). The CNS has an overlap or influence over the ANS and this overlap is used during meditation and other forms of relaxation therapy.

Brain — The brain is the primary organ system of the human being. The brain is the organ system of existence as there is no direct connection between the brain and the "outside" world. The brain coordinates many functions for the purpose of survival and reproduction. The brain creates our existence (awareness) much like a computer simulates "reality" by creating a virtual set of experiences.

Brain States — Brain states are unique conditions that involve level of consciousness, metabolic state, control, and purpose. The brain has two main states: 1. Awake state. 2. Sleep state.

Consolidation of Memory — Memory begins as a biochemical entity. Depending on emotional assignment by the limbic system, memory is transferred from the biochemical form to a structural form. The transformational process from biochemical to structural form is called consolidation of memory.

Cortex — The brain has areas where brain cells are concentrated, i.e., gray matter when viewed in the fresh brain specimen. The cortex of the brain is a surface layer of brain cells called the gray mantel.

Cortical Deactivation — The brain functions during the awake state as a result of cortical activation. The first step in the process to get to sleep is to relax or deactivate the cortex, so that the sleep center can gain control of brain function. Deactivation of the cortex can occur from other processes such as alcoholic intoxication, strokes in midbrain or brain stem, and a whole host of others.

DSMIV — Diagnostic Statistical Manual IV (number four). A book used by psychiatrists to aide in making psychiatric diagnoses. The DSMIV provides behavioral clusters that provide behavioral symptoms that define brain failure (e.g. brain syndromes).

Deactivation of the Cortex — The cortex is activated during the awake state that causes low voltage fast waves. When the cortex is deactivated, control of cortical activity is transferred to the sleep center. The brain wave activity after deactivation, which reflects sleep, is high voltage slow waves. Deactivating the cortex is the transfer of control of cortical activity or control to the sleep center.

Delayed Sleep Phase Syndrome (DSPS) — A disorder in the timing of sleep. Sleep onset is delayed in relationship to desired sleep time. Patient is unable to go to sleep until very late night or early morning. If the patient is required to get up at a normal awake time, he/she will be sleep deprived or tired during the day.

Dyssomnias — A term referring to disorders that involve initiating and maintaining sleep for restorative purposes. Parasomnias are motor sensory or experiential events that occur during sleep.

Electrochemical — The brain is an electrochemical machine. Electric current is produced by brain cells that travel down the axon. At the end of the axon are chemicals that can be released to communicate with the next cell or cells.

Energy and Neurotransmitter Debt — The brain has a reserve of neurotransmitters and energy. When the brain reserve is utilized, it creates a debt. To pay back the debt, energy and neurotransmitter current demands must be met (interest on debt) plus energy and neurotransmitter production to pay back debt (mortgage).

Entrainment — Means to make occur at the same time. In the case of sleep, entrainment means sleep and night time (darkness) occur at the same time.

Histamine — A neurotransmitter that activates the cortex of the brain, mainly in the frontal lobes. Histamine release is controlled by the sleep center via the release of the hormone orexin (hypocrin). During sleep states orexin (and thusly histamine) is turned off which contributes to the deactivation of the cortex.

Hypothalamus — A middle structure of the brain (below the thalamus) which contains a large number of instinctive behaviors. 1. connecting the brain with the body and 2. the measurement of physiological needs.

Kindling — A term that refers to an ever increasing ease of entering an abnormal brain state with each sequential abnormal brain state. An example is the probability of a depressive brain state based on prior episodes of depression.

	Probability of Depression in 5 years
After 1st episode	50%
After 2nd episode	75%
After 3rd episode	90%

L-trytophan — A molecule called an amino acid. Amino acids are molecules that have a amino group and an acid group attached to them. Proteins are a series of attached amino acids that when digested release amino acids for use in the body. One of the uses of L-tryptophan is in the brain. L-tryptophan is converted to seratonin which a neurotransmitter. Seratonin can be converted to melatonin that is a hormone which is related to the timing of sleep with darkness.

Limbic System — A midline structure of the brain that functions to motivate the frontal lobes (DLPC) to plan and execute task to satisfy instincts. The limbic system punishes with negative emotional form of anxiety, guilt and depression.

Mechanisms that activate the frontal lobes (i.e. awake state) — Activation of the brain occurs by three neurotransmitter mechanisms.

Location	Name of Brain cells	Neurotransmitters	Focus of Activation
1. Base of frontal lobes	Basal Nucleus of Meynert	Release of acytlcholine	Hippocampus (memory)
2. Mid-brain	Ventral Tegmental Area	Release of dopamine	Left brain planning executing tasks
3. Brain Stem	Locus cereleus	Release of N:E	Right brain exploratory behavior, associations, creating frontal lobe activation
4. Hypothalamus	Tuboinfidibular nucleus (All nucleus)	Histamine	Related to sleep and activation of frontal lobes (DLPC)

Melatonin — A hormone released by the pineal gland during darkness to coordinate sleep with night time. The retinal/hypothylamic track signals darkness to the pineal gland.

Normal Sleep is sleep that provides for normal behavior during the day, which includes:
1. Self-functioning (how we feel)
2. Social functioning
3. Interpersonal functioning
4. Industrial functioning (work)

Neurotransmitters — Chemicals released from one brain cell that communicates with another brain cell at close range. Distant cells communicate via chemicals called hormones.

Organ System — The human body is built on an organ system model. The brain is the primary organ system which involves awareness, cognitive abilities, ability to plan and execute tasks, ability to coordinate all other organ systems for the purpose of survival (sustain life) and reproduction (sustain species).

Parasomnia — Any undesired motor, verbal or experiential phenomena that occurs during sleep, such as sleep walking.

Periodic Limb Movement of Sleep — Normally, limb movements during sleep are minimal and do not disrupt sleep. Some conditions such as low iron stores can cause limb movement which disrupt sleep. Another condition that causes PLMS is Restless Leg Syndrome, renal dialysis, iron deficiency as reflected in low serum ferritin, and a whole host of others.

Primary Insomnia — A condition due to a weak sleep generator pull to sleep, i.e. caused by primary sleep mechanisms verses secondary to depression or other causes.

Psycho-physiological Insomnia — A term referring to psychological reactions to physiological mechanisms. Psycho-physiological sleep disorder refers to a negative attitude (psychological) that occurs when a person has a physiological reason for not going to sleep. The negative attitude for not going to sleep can in itself be a cause of not being able to go to sleep.

RAS — Reticular Activating System — A diffuse area in the brain system that activates the cortex of the brain during awake state. The sleep center turns off the RAS during sleep.

RLS — Restless Leg Syndrome — A neurological disorder that induces the following symptoms:
1. Urge to get up and move around
2. Involuntary movement of legs which tends to worsen at night
3. Pain in legs which is a very uncomfortable feeling that is partially relieved by rubbing the painful area
4. Disrupted sleep from the above symptoms

Restorative Sleep — Sleep that satisfies three clinical parameters.
1. When a person awakes they feel "rested" (i.e., the hypothalamus is signaling full tank of gas)
2. When a person awakes they feel "well" (i.e., the limbic system rewards the person for satisfying the instinct of sleep by a sense of well-being)

The person with restorative sleep functions normally during the day without signs of sleep deprivation such as tiredness or excessive day-time hypersomnalance.

Reuptake Mechanisms — Brain cells reuse neurotransmitters by pumping them back into the brain cell (i.e., reuptake mechanisms).

Reversal of Circadian Rhythm — The sleep/wake cycle is the circadian rhythm. Normally, humans sleep at night and are awake during the day which is the normal sleep/wake cycle. Reversal of the circadian cycle occurs when a person is awake at nights and sleeps during the day.

Sleep — A unique brain state of the purpose of restoring neurotransmitters and energy reserves to run the brain the next day.

Sleep Center — Several areas of the hypothalamus and brain stem that are involved with initiating, maintaining and providing restorative sleep.

Sleep Debt — In all organ systems there is a reserve or excess capacity. For instance, one can lose an entire lung or kidney and still have normal functioning capacity. The same principle applies to the brain. Part of organ system reserve is the capacity to withstand a temporary period of excess demand that utilizes reserve and creates a metabolic debt. In the case of sleep, loss of reserve and continued inability to provide adequate restorative sleep is called sleep debt.

Sleep Diary — Systematic daily recording of sleep information such as:
1. Time to bed
2. Time to get to sleep
3. Awake time
4. Total hours of sleep
5. Number of awakenings
6. Disturbances during sleep
7. Activities before sleep

8.   Caffeine intake and time
9.   Drugs taken

Sleep Hygiene — Measures taken to enhance sleep such as avoidance of caffeine. Principles of sleep hygiene reinforce normal physiological mechanisms that promote sleep.

Three Steps to Get to Sleep — To get to sleep is a 3-step process of giving up awake control of the brain and giving control of the brain to the sleep center. The three steps are:

Step 1.   Deactivate the cortex
Step 2.   Melatonin key
Step 3.   Pull to sleep by sleep center

Three Steps to Get Restorative Sleep

Step 1.   (Light sleep) transport amino acids into the brain cells.
Step 2.   (Deep sleep) convert amino acids to the neurotransmitter gas.
Step 3.   (REM sleep) deliver gas to the brain engine. Ready the neurotransmitters for release the next day.

Bibliography

American Psychiatric Association: *Diagnostic and Statistical Manual of Mental Disorders*, Fourth Edition, Text Revision, Washington, DC, American Psychiatric Association, 2000. pg. 356.

American Psychiatric Association: *Diagnostic and Statistical Manual of Mental Disorders*, Fourth Edition, Text Revision. Washington, DC, American Psychiatric Association 2000.

American Psychiatric Association: *Diagnostic and Statistical Manual of Mental Disorders*, Fourth Edition, Text Revision Washington, DC, American Psychiatric Association, 2000.

Arch. General Psychiatry 1981; 38:737–746.

Breslau et al. *Biol Psychiatry*, 1996; 39–411.

Camhi SL, Morgan WJ, Pernisco N, Quan SF, Factors affecting sleep disturbances in children and adolescents. *Sleep Med.* 2000; 1:117–123.

Dr. Robert A. Williams' formulation for establishing biological stability of the brain.

Dr. Williams' guess.

DSM IV-TR™ pg. 476.

Haimov I, Lavi P, Landon M, ef Malatonin replacement therapy of the elderly insomniacs. Sleep. 1995; 18:58–603.

Harrison's Principles of Internal Medicine, pg. 212.

Insomnia and Sleep Complaints: What is Normal in the Older Adult? Melinda S. Lantz MD, *Clinical Geriatrics,* Vol. 10, Number 5, May, 2002.

Klink ME, Quan SF, Icaltenborn WT, Lebowitz MR, Risk factors associated with complaints of insomnia in a general white population. *Arch Intern Med.* 1992; 152:1634–1637.

Melatonin, Circadian Rhythms and Sleep, *New England Journal of Medicine* 2000; 343:1114–1116.

New England Journal of Medicine, Vol. 347, No. 7, Pg. 501.

NCSDR/NHTSA Expert Panel on Driver Fatigue and Sleepiness. Drowsy driving and automobiles crashes. Accessed February 22, 2000.

Principles and Practice of Sleep Medicine, 3rd Ed., Kryger Roth Dement, pg. 844.

Principles & Practice of Sleep Medicine, 3rd Ed. Kryger, Roth, Dement, WB Saunders Co., 2002, pg. 694.

Principles & Practice of Sleep Medicine, 3rd Ed. Kryger, Roth, Dement, WB Saunders Co., 2002, pg. 726

Principles & Practice of Sleep Medicine, 3rd Ed. Kryger, Roth, Dement, WB Saunders Co., 2002, pg. 695.

Principles and Practice of Sleep Medicine, Kryger, Roth and Dement, pg. 547.

Principles and Practice of Sleep Medicine by Kryger Roth Dement, WB Saunders Company©2000, pg. 20.

Principals and Practice of Sleep Medicine Third Edition, Kryger, Roth and Dement. Pg. 1140,

Roth T, Roehrs TA, Carkadon MA, Dement WC, Daytime sleepiness and alertness. In: Kryger MH, Roth T, Dement WC, Eds, Principles & Practice of Sleep Medicine. 2nd ed. Philadelphia PA; WB Saunders, 1994; 40–41.

Shift Work, Circadian Disreption and Consequences by Naomi L. Rogers Ph.D. and David F. Dinges, Ph.D., Ten, 2001; 3(9):54–94.

Sleep Medicine, Kryger, Roth & Dement, pg. 1188.